Actual Weight Loss

Mohammed S. Alo, DO

IMPORTANT

If you have a print copy of this book, or someone emailed it to you, it's very important to follow the link below to get on the mailing list to get the free bonus chapters, recipes, workbooks, and any future updates to the book and research studies.

https://DrAlo.net/free

Copyright and Permissions

All copyrights are held by Z Media Group LLC (ZMG) and its subsidiaries. As a ZMG customer, you are permitted to print one (1) copy of this book for your own personal use or read it on a digital device. Such printing may be done by a commercial printer and permission is hereby granted to commercial printers to print this book for the purposes set herein.

You may not email this book or otherwise share it with anyone who has not paid the nominal fee to purchase this book. We have gone out of our way to make this book very affordable and accessible to everyone so that everyone can learn to lose weight properly and benefit from this educational material. The nominal fee helps cover the cost of hosting and delivery of the book to the masses. We take copyright infringements and violations very seriously and will enforce them to the fullest extent of the law. Thank you for your support!

Medical Liability Waiver

I am not your doctor. I do not know you and your medical history personally. I have no idea if you are capable of using the concepts and ideas in this book or in any of Dr. Alo's programs ("Dr. Alo's Content"). **Please talk to your doctor and find out if going on a calorie restricted diet and starting an exercise and fitness program is safe for you!**

If you have an eating disorder, you must see a therapist, especially if you can find one that specializes in eating disorders. The advice in this program would not be beneficial for you and may even exacerbate eating disorders. We cannot be held responsible nor liable for any harm that may occur.

It is strongly recommended that you consult with your physician before beginning any exercise program or making any dietary changes or undertaking any other activities described in this book, on our websites, or in any of Dr. Alo's online and mobile platforms, lectures, PowerPoint presentations, books, webinars, videos, seminars, conferences, podcasts, documents, PDF files, worksheets, cheatsheets, guides, and videos owned and operated by Z Media Group, LLC, Dr. Alo, and his subsidiaries ("Dr. Alo's Content"). You need to be in good physical condition to be able to participate in the diet and exercises described in Dr. Alo's Content including both the diet and exercise programs. You must discuss this with your own doctor and specialists that know you and your medical conditions intimately and personally. Specifically, by accepting these terms and proceeding with Dr. Alo's Content you hereby affirm that you have been cleared by your physician(s), are in good physical condition, and do not suffer from any known physical, emotional, psychological, or mental disability or condition which would prevent or limit your participation in dieting, changing eating habits, vigorous physical activity including but not limited to: resistance training, body weight calisthenics, cardiovascular training, jumping, running, stretching, weight lifting, swimming, walking, jogging, etc. You fully understand that you may severely injure yourself as a result of your enrollment and subsequent participation in any book, course or program that Dr. Alo may recommend and you hereby release ZMG and Dr. Alo and his agents from any and all claims or causes of action, known or unknown, now or in the future related to participating in activities or information described in or arising out of Dr. Alo's Content. These conditions may include, but are not limited to, strokes, heart attacks, muscle strains, muscle pulls, muscle tears, broken bones, shin splints, heat prostration, injuries to knees, injuries to back, injuries to foot, or any other illness or soreness that you may incur, including death and other severe illnesses.

While Dr. Alo is a fully licensed cardiologist and certified personal trainer, he is not your physician nor your personal trainer. He has not assessed you and knowns nothing about you and your medical conditions. He has no ability to diagnose, examine, or treat any of your medical conditions, or in determining the effect of any specific exercise on a medical condition without a personal assessment and full examination which he does not provide online. The information provided by Dr. Alo is not intended to be a substitute for personalized professional medical advice, diagnosis or treatment. You must be examined by your medical team and personal physician before beginning a new diet or exercise program. After attending workshops, conferences, reading articles, watching videos, listening to podcasts (or video audio) or accessing any of Dr. Alo's Content, you are encouraged to review the information carefully with your own professional healthcare provider and personal physician to determine if this is acceptable and safe for you. Never disregard professional medical advice, or delay in seeking medical advice because of something you have learned from Dr. Alo's Content. Never rely on information in Dr. Alo's Content in place of seeking professional medical advice. Dr. Alo is not your physician and is not familiar with your medical and physical condition.

By continuing this program, you agree to release Dr. Alo and any of his subsidiaries of any and all liability.

Contents

Dedication

To my family and friends who have supported me all of these years. And to my patients and clients who encouraged me to write a book for the masses for them to be able to share and read more on true and Actual Weight Loss.

Foreword

Before we get into the meat of this book, I wanted to let you all know that you can find even more information, articles, books, videos, resources, and content on https://DrAlo.net

There are online courses that dive deep into weight loss. There is a one on one coaching program and you can apply to work with me directly at https://DrAlo.net

You can watch all of my health related and weight loss related videos on http://DrAlo.tv

Look out for my calorie-based cookbook for incredibly flavorful, heart healthy, nutritious recipes that add up to your calorie count that's needed for weight loss!

Testimonials

Mo Idlibby, Attorney
Dallas, Texas

I was 240 pounds and I could barely breathe and keep up with my boys. My face was huge, my gut hung out, I had no energy. I couldn't fit into anything anymore. I tried various types of diets over the years. I would lose weight and gain it all back. Over and over again. It was hard! It's been my life since graduating law school. It's embarrassing, because I played Division 1 football at Davidson College and now, I looked like the exact opposite of an athlete.

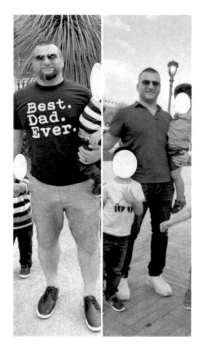

I'm an attorney with a very busy national law firm with multiple offices in different states and I have 4 young children, I had no time for anything. Literally, no time to even sit down. I was building my business and practice. I had no time to go to the gym, no time to work out. Dr. Alo showed me that I don't need time to make these simple changes.

I was desperate. I was defeated. I threw a Hail Mary and reached out to Dr. Alo hoping he could help. I was trying to do keto at the time, the fifth time I had tried it. Dr. Alo counseled me on the phone and through video and we got a plan together. Keto works a little, then I kept gaining the weight back. I was tired of it. I needed an end game. A way to finally beat obesity.

I followed Dr. Alo's plan precisely and I got down to 175 pounds! And have kept it off for two years now! And because of the education and teaching, this will be my new way of living. I can eat pretty much whatever I want, and I can still lose weight.

Thank you Dr. Alo!

Anurag Tandon, Businessman
Naperville, IL

Although I was athletic during high school and in my early 20s, my weight ballooned, and my health declined in my 30s and 40s. This was due to making unhealthy lifestyle choices. I would consume sugary drinks at every meal, hard to say no to dessert and eat fast food multiple times a week. One day I became embarrassed by the person I was seeing in pictures. I had become a bit of a running joke amongst my friends regarding my stomach and ability to eat so much at one meal.

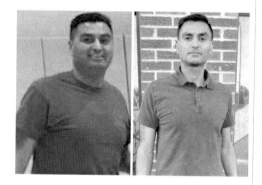

I had tried lifting weights off and on for nearly a decade with little to no visible results. But when I started to follow Dr. Alo's advice regarding healthy food choices and developing a healthy relationship with food - I finally began to see the positive changes I knew I could achieve. Based entirely on Dr. Alo's advice I was able to lose 40 lbs in five months and get stronger.

The most important part of my journey was the confidence I now have with food. I know that is okay to eat what I want. I know that if I gain weight that I can take it off. I know what to look for and how to fit it in to my food choices. Dr. A helped me look nearly 10 years younger. I'm stronger and more muscular, I feel energized and am super excited about the life I have created. If I can shave years off my life - you can also.

With love,
Anurag Tandon

Melissa Spieker
Deerfield, Illinois

I've always loved sports and have always been an athlete. But then I became a mom and everything changed. I had no time to do anything. My body changed. I tried every fad diet known to man and I was stuck. I would lose a few pounds, and then not know what to do. I couldn't get

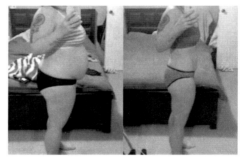

back to my original weight (or even close). My weight ballooned and my health declined in my 30s. Now, I have 3 kids. I tried every fad diet there was and just couldn't maintain weight loss. I was eating only 1200 calories and in the gym daily doing the stair climber, running on treadmills, and doing all kinds of things. Weight just wouldn't come off.

I had a terrible relationship with food. Every food was "bad" or "good" and I could never stick to my diet.

One day I became embarrassed by the person I was seeing in the mirror. I couldn't fit into my jeans. I lost my confidence. I stopped caring. I wore baggy clothes just to hide.

Then I finally met Dr. Alo. I started to follow Dr. Alo's advice regarding healthy food choices and developing a healthy relationship with food. I was in tears. I didn't realize how bad my relationship with food and exercise was. Dr. Alo taught me not to punish myself in the gym and with food. I learned to enjoy, take days off, have diet breaks, improve my mental health and self-care. All while still losing

12

weight, getting better definition, and improving my confidence. I know I can eat whatever I want, whenever I want and still maintain or lose weight. If I gain weight, I just shave it off. I'm so grateful!

With Dr. Alo's help I look nearly 20 years younger, I am stronger, leaner, I feel more confident and am happier than I have ever been (and I can actually keep up with my kids!) If I can reverse 20 years of bad habits - you can too!"

Thank you so much!
Melissa Speiker

Chapter 1

Introduction

"Yikes!"

I was 39 years old and looking at a picture I had just taken at work with my staff. I was basically obese. Yes, obese. I couldn't believe it. I was absolutely obese! I was just about to turn 40. I was fit and athletic. I still played basketball and soccer every week, but I was still obese. And up until a few years ago, when I was 37, I still played tackle football.

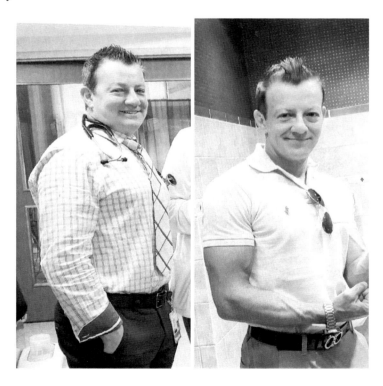

How can this be? How can "The Weight Loss Doctor" be obese? What have I done? And what can I do about it?

I was devastated. You know the feeling of defeat? When you think you are doing everything right, but you fail miserably? That's how I felt. After all these years of preaching about weight loss, I actually lost… to weight loss.

I first began lecturing on healthy living, fitness, and weight loss when I was in high school. I spoke mainly about fitness, and I preached how anyone should be able to lose weight, making small changes to their lifestyle.

When I first started high school, I was 117 pounds, and just barely got to 155 by the time I graduated. At 5 foot 8 inches, that was not a bad weight. After a year or two of college, I was 193 and almost the heaviest I have ever been. I even bragged about being 193 when I was playing basketball with friends at the University of Toledo's brand new $30 million dollar rec center, banging bodies under the rim! Uggg!

Don't get me wrong, to most people I probably didn't look "obese". But I was. And I was not happy with myself. I was very disappointed.

I did what most people would do and started following the latest fad diet. At that time, the Atkins Diet was popular (and written by a doctor) so I decided to do it.

After an agonizing 8 months, I got down to 168 pounds. But I didn't look good at all. I was "skinny fat". Sure, the scale showed less weight, but the mirror told a different story.

Skinny fat is when a man or woman weighs a lot less, but still carry around a lot of body fat and still don't look very toned or muscular.

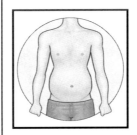

A few years later. Dr Agaston (a cardiologist who invented the cardiac CT scan) came out with a book called the South Beach Diet. It was like Atkins, but you ate healthier fats, proteins, and carbs. People in South Beach, Florida (where he is based) were doing it and having good results. I tried that too and lost a few pounds and then gained it all back.

A friend of mine at the time gave me the Sugarbusters diet book and I tried that. I lost a few pounds then gained it back.

Fast forward to medical school. I was hovering between 178 and 193 pounds, but never lower. It was frustrating. I was healthy, fit, athletic, played every sport, but was quite overweight. I even published a diet book in 2006 called, The Alo Diet. And people loved it, but it was also unsustainable and only caused short term results. It was a low carb, high protein style diet. It worked, but no one could do it long enough. Obviously, we know a lot more about diet and nutrition now.

Over the years, I would try nearly every diet there was. I bought and read every diet book and learned a lot. Science was fascinating to me. I wanted to know why these diets worked or didn't work. Sure, I learned a lot, but I would still end up overweight.

Why?

That's the part I couldn't figure out. Why did it work for a bit, then I end up overweight again? It was very frustrating to me. I needed a better way. Especially, since I was lecturing on weight loss and teaching other physicians about weight loss. I needed to figure this out fast!

I did eventually figure it out, and that's why I decided to write this book. I don't want anyone else to have to go through what I had to go through to figure it out. This can be your "cheat code" or shortcut to safe, effective, and permanent weight loss that doesn't rely on fads and gimmicks. (And you can eat whatever you want! Shhhh!)

Coming Together

Fast forward to 2018. I was 197 pounds now, nearly a year after having reconstructive knee surgery to repair my torn ACL. The ACL didn't slow me down or cause me to gain weight, my weight was holding steady from before and after knee surgery. I was hovering between 183 and 197. I was at my highest. That's when that picture above was taken.

I decided to post a challenge on Facebook and have people do it with me. My goal was to do 100 pushups and 100 squats per day for 30 days. I called it #AloChallenge and people did it with me. At first, I could only do 10-15 pushups in a row, but could do almost all 100 bodyweight squats without stopping. My legs had always been strong because I had played football for so long. Eventually, I was able to do about 60 pushups in a row. But I was still fat.

Yes, after a month of exercise and strength training, I was still overweight. I was shocked. But now I know why. More on this later.

By spring of 2018, my wife had joined a gym and started working out with trainers. I had a small home gym so I started lifting weights at home to show that I can do it too. Nothing changed for me at all. But my wife did see some initial benefits (more on why this doesn't sustain past a few months later), but she gained it all back.

In August of 2018, I decided to have that trainer come to my house and train me. He did. I got stronger and he wore me out. But I was still fat. He eventually moved to Charlotte, North Carolina to play college football.

My wife had changed gyms and she hired a different trainer. He was training her well and she was getting stronger. So, in October of 2018, I signed up with him and decided I needed to do this right.

He had me bench pressing, squatting, deadlifting, and doing all the right compound movements and I was definitely getting stronger. Finally?

No. By January of 2019, I was still overweight, and my trainer moved away. So, I researched body building and started training myself. I actually got much stronger, and my main lifts all went up. I stopped doing some of the crazier "Instagram Worthy" stuff that he had me doing, and I enjoyed lifting weights. I got very strong.

"There's no point in bench pressing 300 pounds if you also weigh 300 pounds".

I said this to myself a few times. I didn't want to be that guy that could bench 300 pounds and also weighed 300 pounds. I was frustrated.

The Journey Begins

This is when my real weight loss and fitness journey began. For years now, all I did was frustrate myself and not achieve my goals.

I turned to the fitness and bodybuilding industry. If anyone knew how to lose weight and get ripped, it was them. Men and women.

I started watching videos, reading articles, and ordered nearly every book on fitness and bodybuilding you can imagine. And yes, I read them all. Nearly 40 books (and over $1000 dollars). I also watched hundreds, if not thousands of YouTube videos on bodybuilding. I even hired multiple coaches that prepare people for bodybuilding shows. I was thirsty for knowledge, and I wanted it all!

After all this research, I realized I was missing the "eating right" part of fitness. You must eat in a way to support your goals. I was not doing that. I wasn't tracking or eating any differently at all. So, I decided to start tracking. This may sound obvious to some of you, but it wasn't obvious to me. Sure, I was eating healthy. I didn't eat processed foods, never ate fast food, and only ate home cooked, wholesome meals. But I was still fat. Yes, you can gain weight eating healthy, more on that later.

January 21, 2019, I decided to go on a 1400 calorie a day diet and supplemented with some whey protein daily to hit at least 100g of protein per day. Knowing what I know now, that was not the best idea. But I didn't know any better. More on this later. But I thought this should work.

Fourteen hundred calories a day, for an active male weighing 195 pounds is a very low calorie count. It was not the best decision, but that's what I knew at the time.

In March 2019, I decided that I wanted to be a personal trainer, so I researched and decided to do the NASM course and become certified. On May 24, 2019, I took my exam and passed. It was a great education, and perfect to pair with cardiology. It gave me a whole new perspective on health and fitness and my patients and students (other doctors) benefitted tremendously from my newfound knowledge.

Back to my 1400 calorie diet. It worked. I was super strict. I used MyFitnessPal to track every morsel. I bought a food scale and even weighed every "green grape" I would put in my mouth. I even bought a small, portable food scale to take to work with me. I was so strict that I would go out to dinner with my parents and only order water and watched them all eat, because "I was out of calories" for the day. Was it crazy? Yes! But it also worked. Sometimes you have to be a little crazy to achieve your goals! (I wouldn't do it this way again, by the way. I had a very bad relationship with food).

By August 15, 2019, I was down to 145 pounds. Yes, 145! The lowest I had weighed since I was maybe 16 or 17 years old. I had lost 50 pounds! My body fat percentage was 7%. Yes, seven percent! Single digits! Lean enough to step on stage at a bodybuilding show and win an award. Of course, I didn't do this, I don't think people want to see their cardiologist prancing around on stage half naked!

It was weird. People asked me if I had cancer, if I was sick, if anything was wrong? My answer was, "No, I'm just trying to lose weight".

It worked, and it worked well! It was glorious! I finally did it!

Or did I?

Right after that, I hired another body building nutrition coach and he told me everything that I had done wrong. I knew it wasn't perfect. But, yeah, I did it wrong. So, now I know. I changed a lot of things.

He told me I should increase my calories and go on a bulk. So, starting September 2019, I decided to eat more and bulk back up. Still lifting weights nearly every day, I got up to 178 maybe 183 pounds by January 2020. I know I got bigger and stronger. But I needed to figure out what to do next.

So, I hired another coach who spent 3 months coaching me properly back down to 163. I was ripped and shredded again, but had way more muscle this time. Because I was actually doing it right. I ate the correct amount of calories (not 1400) and ate enough protein. Both on the way up when bulking, and on the way back down again when cutting weight.

My conversations with this coach were endless. We talked for hours. Obviously, I paid him a lot of money. You have to be willing to invest in yourself and your education. And I did.

Now I felt like I had finally arrived. I would go on to start coaching friends and family on proper weight loss and nutrition and they were all seeing tremendous results. Whether they wanted to get stronger, leaner, tone up, just lose weight, gain muscle, whatever their fitness goals were, I was able to help them.

I am in a lot of fitness and health groups on Facebook, GroupMe, and WhatsApp and it has been really inspiring to watch people lose weight the right way. I have had some people lose upwards of 120 pounds or more all following a simple plan that doesn't require any crazy food restrictions. They are eating whatever they want, and losing tons of weight! It's so humbling and satisfying! I receive thousands of messages a day telling me how thankful and grateful they are for meeting me and following my plan.

What Does Bodybuilding Have to Do With You?

You may be thinking to yourself, "I'm not a bodybuilder, nor do I ever want to be, how is this going to help me"?

After reading hundreds of books on weight loss, fitness, and bodybuilding, and reading nearly every single research study on weight loss, and after spending thousands of dollars on coaching and education, I decided to break this all down into a simple to follow plan so that you don't have to spend thousands of dollars. You have this book, it's cheap and it has everything in it you will ever need! You already invested in this book, you don't need to spend thousands to hire coaches or pay for anything else!

No, you don't have to be a bodybuilder to lose weight. You don't have to want any of that. You can lose weight and just look like an ordinary person. You may even want to just look "skinny fat". And that's ok. But you may start losing weight and like your results and want to get pretty shredded and pretty lean. When I finally got below 173 pounds, I decided to keep going because I saw more lines and more muscles. When I got to 165, I did the same. Even more lines. When I got to 151, I was at 8% body fat, but I wanted to push myself and go further. Finally, I got to 145 and stopped. It was enough. I was the leanest I had ever been and looked pretty ripped. But I was also too small. I looked like a 12 year old little boy. I knew this wasn't right either.

No one can tell you what to do or how to look. Only you get to decide that. You can get as lean as you want, or as big as you want. No one can decide but you.

With all of that said, let me take you on this journey and let me show you and teach you everything that I've learned along the way, so you don't have to struggle and pay so much out of pocket to learn all of this!

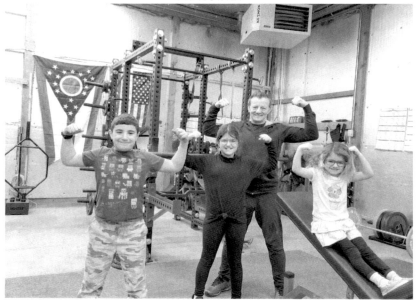

This is a picture of me and my kids working out together in my home gym. Establishing good habits from an early age is crucial to altering human behavior and changing long term priorities.

Human Behavior

A lot of what we will be discussing in this book is not just the research and science of weight loss, but how it applies to human behavior. For example, you could just eat fat and protein and lose a lot of weight, but that won't be very sustainable. I'm sure most of you have tried that, I know I did. Another example would be jogging 6 miles per day. Sure, you could lose a lot of weight doing that, but you can't do that for the next 50 years. (Your knees will hate you!)

Part of my job as a cardiologist and a personal trainer is to teach people behavior patterns, frameworks, and mindsets that promote a healthy relationship with food and a healthy relationship with exercise. I also want to promote relationships that are sustainable long term. You must select a diet and exercise strategy that you can adhere to for the rest of your life. And you must select a framework and behavior pattern that you can adhere to for the rest of your life.

The goal of this book will be to incorporate the science of weight loss with what we know about human behavior and sustainability. While something may work for weight loss, we want to make sure it sustainable and not causing new eating disorders or long-term weight regain.

Chapter 2

Scope of the Obesity Problem

In 2021
- 82% of adults overweight
- 22% of adults obese
- 18% of children 2-19 years of age are overweight (5.6% Obese)
- 12% of children 2-5 years of age are overweight

You've all seen these charts and graphs before. Below is the first chart comparing obesity rates in 1994, 1996, to 2004 for adults. Notice that by 2004, they had to use new colors to depict states that had obesity rates over 25%

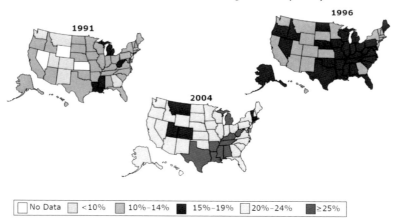

Obesity Trends* Among U.S. Adults
BRFSS, 1991, 1996, 2004
(*BMI ≥30, or about 30 lbs overweight for 5'4" person)

| | No Data | <10% | 10%–14% | 15%–19% | 20%–24% | ≥25% |

And by 2011, now there are even more orange states depicting obesity rates over 30%, see below.

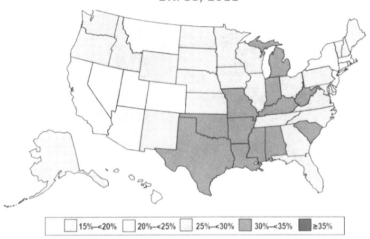

Prevalence of Self-Reported Obesity Among U.S. Adults
BRFSS, 2011

15%–<20%   20%–<25%   25%–<30%   30%–<35%   ≥35%

Now look at the 2016-2018 chart below. There are even more dark, maroon-colored states depicting obesity rates over 35%. And the orange is obesity rates of 30-35%. The darker maroon states have nearly taken over.

Prevalence of Self-Reported Obesity Among Non-Hispanic Black Adults by State and Territory, BRFSS, 2016-2018

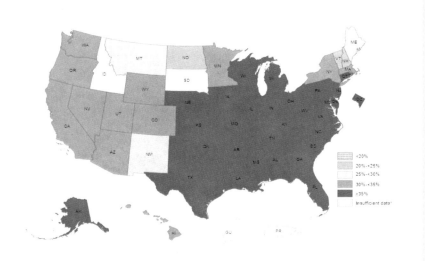

In the chart below, you see that overweight men and women have held steady since the 1960s. However, obesity and extreme obesity rates have gone up significantly.

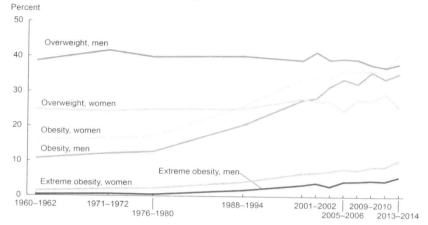

Figure. Trends in adult overweight, obesity, and extreme obesity among men and women aged 20–74: United States, 1960–1962 through 2013–2014

NOTES: Age-adjusted by the direct method to the year 2000 U.S. Census Bureau estimates using age groups 20–39, 40–59, and 60–74. Overweight is body mass index (BMI) of 25 kg/m² or greater but less than 30 kg/m²; obesity is BMI greater than or equal to 30; and extreme obesity is BMI greater than or equal to 40. Pregnant females were excluded from the analysis.
SOURCES: NCHS, National Health Examination Survey and National Health and Nutrition Examination Surveys.

What's more alarming is the increase in childhood obesity rates, take a look below.

What are the trends in adult and childhood obesity?

From 1999–2000 through 2015–2016, a significantly increasing trend in obesity was observed in both adults and youth. The observed change in prevalence between 2013–2014 and 2015–2016, however, was not significant among both adults and youth (Figure 5).

Figure 5. Trends in obesity prevalence among adults aged 20 and over (age adjusted) and youth aged 2–19 years: United States, 1999–2000 through 2015–2016

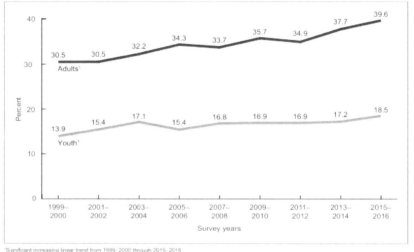

¹Significant increasing linear trend from 1999–2000 through 2015–2016.
NOTES: All estimates for adults are age adjusted by the direct method to the 2000 U.S. census population using the age groups 20–39, 40–59, and 60 and over. Access data table for Figure 5 at: https://www.cdc.gov/nchs/data/databriefs/db288_table.pdf#5.
SOURCE: NCHS, National Health and Nutrition Examination Survey, 1999–2016.

Overall Trends

In 1980, 46% of US adults age 20 and older were overweight or obese; by 1999, the number had increased to 60%. This dramatic increase has coincided with several trends:

• Higher energy intake from larger portion at home and at restaurants ("super-sizing")

• Greater consumption of high-fat, higher calorie foods

• Widespread availability of low-cost, good-tasting, energy-dense (high calorie) foods

• Decreased physical activity at work, at home, and during leisure time.

At any given time, 44% of women and 29% of men are dieting.

Americans spend $60 billion a year on weight-loss products, programs, and pills that do absolutely nothing for them. We are still overweight, even more so than before. Gym memberships are up significantly since the 1980s, yet we are still overweight.

Take a look at this graph:

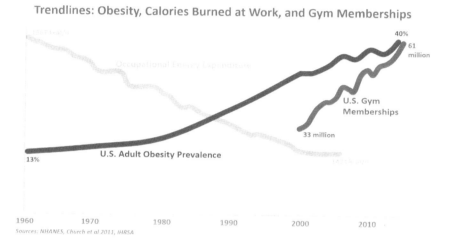

Notice the red and yellow lines. Since the 1960s, obesity has increased while activity and energy expenditure (calories) burned at work has been reduced. We no longer have such labor intense jobs, most jobs are now desk jobs and hard labor is not as common.

The dark blue line denotes gym memberships and shows that those have also been increasing at a rate commensurate with obesity rates.

So while we realize we have a problem, we think that that joining a gym will solve it. We think we can exercise off our calories. Or run them off. Or swim them off. Or bike them off. Or lift them off.

Unfortunately, it just doesn't work that way.

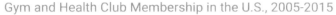

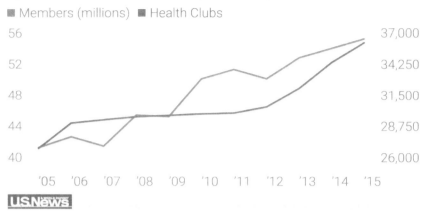

In the above graph, you'll notice that people are still joining gyms and memberships are still increasing.

And the next graphs shows that the gym and fitness industry is quite recession proof.

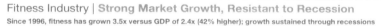

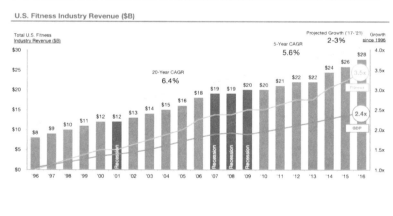

With that being said, we are all still quite overweight and we need the right solution. Telling people to just exercise and start diets isn't going to solve anything. They have tried that and we have tried that. And here we are today, still overweight. More overweight!

Diet Success Rates

Unfortunately, we haven't had much success with diets. The statistics are overwhelming in favor of weight regain. I struggled with this myself over and over again. I would start a "diet", lose weight, then regain it all back, and sometimes more.

As a country….

50-70% weight regain rates in year 1
85% within 2 years
95% in 3 years
33-66% will add back more wight than they lost

But 5% of people lose weight and keep it off past 5 years!

And we will learn how to become part of that 5% and not gain the weight back!

Costs of Obesity?

The numbers are staggering, here's just a few examples. As a country, we could actually save so much money, time, and energy, if we found better ways to help people to lose weight. These numbers are from 2016, it's much worse now!

Q: What is the cost of obesity?
A: Total cost: $147 billion , Direct cost: $65 billion,* Indirect cost: $56 billion (comparable to the economic costs of cigarette smoking)

Q: What is the cost of heart disease related to overweight and obesity?
A: Direct cost: $8.8 billion (17 percent of the total direct cost of heart disease, independent of stroke)

Q: What is the cost of type 2 diabetes related to overweight and obesity?

A: Total cost: $98 billion (in 2001)

Q: What is the cost of osteoarthritis related to overweight and obesity?

A: Total cost: $21.2 billion, Direct cost: $5.3 billion, Indirect cost: $15.9 billion

Q: What is the cost of hypertension (high blood pressure) related to overweight and obesity?

A: Direct cost: $4.1 billion (17 percent of the total cost of hypertension)

Q: What is the cost of gallbladder disease related to overweight and obesity?

A: Total cost: $3.4 billion, Direct cost: $3.2 billion, Indirect cost: $187 million

Q: What is the cost of cancer related to overweight and obesity?

- Breast cancer: Total cost: $2.9 billion, Direct cost: $1.1 billion, Indirect cost: $1.8 billion
- Endometrial cancer: Total cost: $933 million, Direct cost: $310 million, Indirect cost: $623 million
- Colon cancer: Total cost: $3.5 billion, Direct cost: $1.3 billion, Indirect cost: $2.2 billion

Q: What is the cost of lost productivity related to obesity?

- The cost of lost productivity related to obesity (BMI $\geq$ 30) among Americans ages 17–64 is $3.9 billion. This value considers the following annual numbers (for 1994):
- Workdays lost related to obesity: 39.3 million
- Physician office visits related to obesity: 62.7 million
- Restricted activity days related to obesity: 239.0 million
- Bed-days related to obesity: 89.5 million

Medical Complications of Obesity

I'm sure this goes without say, but here's a visual representation of the most common health ailments that are associated with obesity. And there are literally hundreds more. Obesity causes inflammation, and inflammation affects every organ system.

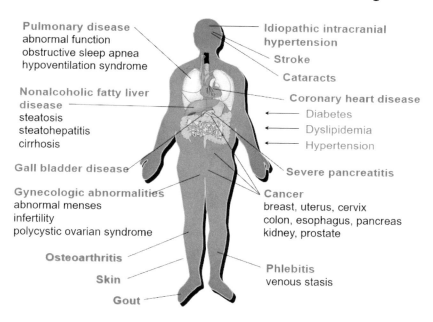

Medical Complications of Obesity

Pulmonary disease
abnormal function
obstructive sleep apnea
hypoventilation syndrome

Idiopathic intracranial hypertension

Stroke

Cataracts

Nonalcoholic fatty liver disease
steatosis
steatohepatitis
cirrhosis

Coronary heart disease

Diabetes

Dyslipidemia

Hypertension

Gall bladder disease

Severe pancreatitis

Gynecologic abnormalities
abnormal menses
infertility
polycystic ovarian syndrome

Cancer
breast, uterus, cervix
colon, esophagus, pancreas
kidney, prostate

Osteoarthritis

Skin

Phlebitis
venous stasis

Gout

Complications of Obesity that No One Ever Talks About

- Not fitting in CT scanner or MRI machine
- Abdominal surgery and healing, can't close back up
- Medical emergencies- Can they carry you out?
- Difficulty dosing medications
- Operating tables not capable
- Not fitting in airplane
- Stress testing equipment can't handle more weight
- Two day tests instead of one

- Inability to draw blood
- Can't fit in certain masks
- Can't be intubated properly
- Not being able to dose medications properly because they were never tested in such large individuals with large volumes of distribution (we don't know if it's even working for you)
- Need specialized heavy equipment to turn patients in hospital beds
- Immobility and bed sores

Energy Balance?

If you look at the scale below, you'll see the balance between energy intake and energy expenditure. While it's true that this is the crux of the problem, there's a lot more nuance to it and a lot more that we need to take into consideration than just this energy balance equation.

But yes, for most people, if your intake is less than your expenditure, you should lose weight. Obviously, it's not that easy, otherwise everyone would be doing it.

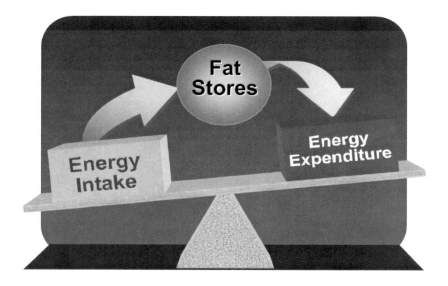

The Dunning Kruger Effect

I am sure you have seen this in action. You find an influencer or one of your friends who starts talking about "I just read this book, and here is the **ONLY** way to lose weight". I used to do this too when I was younger and did not know as much (and didn't know that I didn't know). It's very easy to get caught up in one book or one study that showed x result. We want to look at the totality of evidence and look at the totality of studies. Not just one single source.

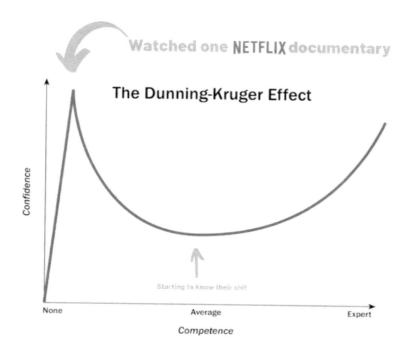

Dunning Kruger

This chart explains the Dunning Kruger Effect beautifully. When you don't know very much, you are less competent, but you are super confident (because you watched that one Netflix documentary). As your knowledge base grows, you are more competent, but begin to realize how little you actually know, so your confidence begins to dip. As you learn even more, you really begin to know more and your confidence begins to go back up. Once you become and expert, your competence is back up as it should be!

So why do people think they know so much after watching one documentary or reading one research article? Is it because an expert wrote it? Was it convincing? Yes, it can sound very authoritative sometimes. They can easily cherry pick studies and research and make it sound so believable. People sometimes don't know any better and listen to experts and believe them, because they themselves, know so little. And experts sound so convincing!

But a lot of times these experts are selling an agenda or an angle. Sure, you could lose weight doing Intermittent Fasting. It can work if certain criteria are met. But that's not the *ONLY* way to lose weight.

An example would be Dr. Jason Fung, a nephrologist from Canada. He wrote a book called The Obesity Code where he discusses intermittent fasting and how it's the best and *ONLY* way to lose weight. He claims that "calories in versus calories out doesn't work". And he tries to cite studies that show this doesn't work. Unfortunately, the studies he cites, didn't even control for calories at all. But far more egregious than that, is his contention that there is no other way to lose weight.

My problem with this, is that it's simply not true. There are so many different ways to lose weight. There is not one right answer. Sure, you could lose weight doing intermittent fasting, or keto, or paleo, or Atkin's or Dash, Jenny Craig, Weight Watchers, Carnivore, Nutrisystem, TB12, Whole 30, and hundreds of other diets. But to claim that there is only one way to lose weight, is simply wrong.

People believe in diets like they are religions. They literally feel shaken to their core if you contradict them. You must be very careful with how you approach people and their "diet religion". If you are talking to a keto believer, they will attack you if you tell them there are other ways to lose weight. You don't have to approach them at all. But once people notice how much weight you have lost, you will become the de facto weight loss expert and they will just come to you and start asking you questions. Just be gentle, kind, humble, and teach!

Chapter 3

Story Time: Pool Party

I was at a pool party last year. Since I'm also a cardiologist, a friend of mine asked me about an episode where he passed out. He passed out driving home from the gym one day and totaled his car and hit three other cars. No one was hurt. But he was shocked and wanted answers. He was young and healthy.

I asked him what he was doing. He said he was doing intermittent fasting and had not drank enough that day, drank some coffee, went to the gym and did a high intensity interval training work out. He said it was very intense. He was lightheaded and dizzy and tried to drive home. Then found himself in a ditch surrounded by paramedics and was taken to the hospital.

He was very dehydrated and hadn't been eating nor drinking much that day and did a very intense work out. And that's what led to his near-death experience. Thankfully, no one was hurt.

I asked him why he was doing intermittent fasting and what was his goal. He is 5 foot 8 inches and weighed 240 pounds. He said he was just trying to lose weight, and someone told him this would work very well. I asked him how long he had been doing this for and he said, "Three months". I asked, "Have you lost weight?" He replied, "No, I gained almost ten pounds."

He nearly killed himself doing intermittent fasting and hadn't lost weight. In fact, he gained weight. This is anecdotal and just one person, but it illustrates that not every diet works for everyone. You must find something that works for you. Don't do what your friends are doing or what's popular. There is a much better way that works for everyone.

One of the other doctors at the pool party looked at him and told him, "Why don't you just eat 1200 calories a day. You'll lose weight if you do that." All my friends looked at me and I sighed and went into teaching mode, teaching about weight loss and proper calorie counts. This happens nearly every day. People know I am "The Weight Loss Doctor" and expect me to dispel all myths and educate on every occasion. I oblige because I love teaching and I enjoy it. Plus, I really didn't want my friend to die!

A 240 pound male eating 1200 calories per day would be very, very hungry. Starving really! And likely won't be getting enough protein. Sure, he would lose weight really fast, but too fast! Losing weight too fast will cause muscle loss. You want to lose weight gradually, so you don't lose muscle. We will dive deep into this topic later. He could also end up very depleted and pass out again. Which we want to avoid.

Who Am I?

I get this question a lot. "Dr. Alo, why should I listen to you? How do you know so much about weight loss?"

I grew up in Toledo, Ohio, played high school football for St. John's Jesuit High School and walked on to my hometown university's Division 1 college football team. My college football career never amounted to anything more than a practice squad dummy, but it was a lot of fun! When the pre-medical classes got hard, I had to drop my football playing dreams.

I studied economics in college. Economics is the study of decision making. Yes, you use it every day. When you are deciding when to fill up gas, you are an economist! When you are deciding what cake to buy, you are an economist! When you are deciding how to cut your hair, you are an economist! Everything is economics! All day, every day!

I didn't know this at the time, but economics would pair very well with cardiology and medicine. And it would also pair very well with weight loss research evaluation and coaching patients and clients on proper weight loss. So many times, you're comparing two different studies and making decisions about which one is more valuable and which one was done better and that's when you have economics coming into play.

Shortly after high school, I began my lecturing career. It started out by lecturing at grade schools about health and fitness. As I finished college and was more educated, I began lecturing at high schools and other venues. When I was in graduate school studying HIV and trying to get into medical school, I would also go back and lecture at local high schools and local societies on HIV.

One of my medical school research projects was about obesity and weight loss in minority populations. I would go on to design a diet and write a book about weight loss called The Alo Diet while still a medical student. People did this diet and loved it and it had a huge following on the internet. At one point, the Facebook group for the Alo Diet had over 20,000 followers. People were posting success stories and transformations every day and it was very inspiring.

Other medical colleges were calling my medical school and asking them to send me over to speak and give presentations at their medical school on obesity and weight loss. So, I would travel the country lecturing on obesity and weight loss. Obviously, I didn't know as much as I know now, but I've always believed that if you know something you should teach it, even if it may not be complete or 100% accurate. People can still learn and be inspired to seek more knowledge.

Once I became a fully licensed physician, I started giving all kinds of lectures at continuing medical education (CME) conferences. Mainly, I would lecture on medical topics and cardiac topics. One day, I commented to one of the organizers that I have a very long lecture on weight loss, they jumped on the opportunity right away and I ended up presenting my two-hour lecture on weight loss. At first, they didn't want to give me two hours. They said that was very long and no one could pay attention for that long on one topic. I proved them wrong! I gave my lecture and when it was all said and done, I received a standing ovation. They literally loved every second of it and not a single person walked out of the room or played on their phone! (I'm a bit of a comedian when I speak too.)

I've always been a very gifted speaker and I can captivate audiences and explain very complex topics in very simple terms. Can you imagine sitting in a room for two hours listening to someone speak on weight loss? That's exactly what I did! Over and over and over again! It became my most requested talk! I've traveled the world teaching physicians how to teach their patients to lose weight. It's a topic I spent the last 20 years diving into and researching. I've read every book and every research article ever published on weight loss, so I truly know what I'm talking about (humble brag).

I've also been through that journey multiple times. My entire life I've been somewhat overweight and even obese. I know the struggles that people go through. I know why people latch on to fads and latch onto crazy diets because they just want to believe in something and hope that something works.

I've had patients cry in my exam rooms telling me that no one ever sat down with them and told them that they need to lose weight. I had other patients start tearing up and crying because I'm the only physician that actually sat down with them and told them how to actually lose weight and didn't sound crazy. It's very sad but it's also very eye opening. Obesity is a huge problem and it's getting worse and worse. It's growing, pun intended.

Smoking cigarettes is the number one cause of heart attacks and strokes. If you smoke, your chance of having a heart attack or stroke is 20 times higher than if you didn't. The next worse thing is obesity. Obesity raises your chance of having heart attack or stroke 10 times normal. Only 19% of this country smokes now, so it's our duty to make sure we get the obesity rates down. Currently about 82% of adults are overweight, 42% are obese, and nearly 20% of children are overweight. This is a huge problem! Once again, pun intended!

As time went on, I would go on to manage multiple health and fitness groups online teaching people how to lose weight properly, for absolutely free! Literally free! Nothing in return. I love this and enjoy it! I don't want your money! I am wealthy beyond anything I could have ever imagined as a son of immigrants growing up. I am living the American Dream and I love every aspect of my life. I love teaching and helping people lose weight. I'm the guy at the gym that picks up the weights of the random stranger and puts them back. I stop on the highway risking my own life to help save yours. I don't need anything. So why do I do this?

I wanted to leave something behind for others to be able to use if I were to disappear. That's why I am writing this book and giving it away for peanuts. I want it to be part of my legacy. I want it to live on after I die. Till after death.

That's the same reason I post my lectures on YouTube, so that others may learn, long after I am gone. I want my students, kids, friends, family, and loved ones to be able to watch me and live through my voice and my advice. I want them to see my sincerity and my mannerisms. I want people to still learn after I am gone. I spent my entire adult life learning this and teaching this, I don't want it to go away with me!

I've had so many physicians and friends tell me to put my lectures and talks on YouTube and I have. Click the text to see my channel. More topics are being added daily.

What Drives Me?

Madness.

The thing that drives me is all the madness that you see online and on social media. If you go through your Facebook feed or Instagram or Tiktok or any other social media platform, you will see hundreds, if not thousands, of different crazy ways to lose weight. Some of them will work, but a lot of them are just fads, gimmicks, and some are just plain dangerous. A lot of these people are selling a false hope or selling very expensive programs. You don't have to pay thousands and thousands of dollars for someone to help you lose weight. You don't have to pay thousands of dollars for a nutrition coach or registered dietitian or a cardiologist or a personal trainer to help you lose weight. This is why I wrote this book! So that you can buy this book for very little and have everything you need to lose weight! It's literally that simple.

My goal for you is to read this book, do some of the exercises in the workbook and workshop part of it, and start to lose weight and never look back. You will lose all the weight you want, and more, if you want to, without doing any crazy diets or anything dangerous. You will eat the food that you love and eat the things that you like and still lose weight. And if you want to look lean, toned, or muscular you can do that too! Everything is in the book!

My Wife and The Inspiration

I was sitting on the couch one night watching a movie with the kids. My wife looked at me and said, "Hey Jenna wants to know what she should do". She hands me her phone so that I could read what Jenna had wrote. Jenna was in one of many WhatsApp groups with my wife, and the topic of weight loss had come up. So, my wife did what she always does and asks me the questions so that I can answer them. But this time she just handed me the phone and I answered all of Jenna's questions. That took over an hour to do. It wasn't very efficient. My wife looked at me and said, "Why don't you write a book or create a course or something so that people can just read it and figure out how to lose weight properly. Aren't you sick of answering questions in all these groups and online when you could just write a book and answer all these questions once?"

That's when it clicked! She gave me the idea to write this book and create online materials and courses for people to read and go through to learn how to lose weight properly. I've seen way too many disasters and way too many people lose a lot of weight quickly and then gain it all back. I've also seen too many people follow dangerous advice and get very sick. What's worse, is many of them would gain back more weight than when they first started. That's when I decided to start making online courses and products and writing this book to help people lose weight the right way. After all I think I'm the only cardiologist out there that's also a certified personal trainer. And I'm probably the only one that has spent over 20 years researching and lecturing on obesity and weight loss. I technically could write the book on weight loss. I guess that's what I just did.

Weight Loss Research

There are lots of ways to study weight loss. One of the best ways to study weight loss is something called a Metabolic Ward Study. You put people into a hospital ward, control everything they eat and don't eat and monitor their weight, basic metabolic rate, and everything that goes in and out very precisely by using something called doubly labelled water. They are expensive, because you have to pay participants a lot of money to take them away from their lives and families for 12 weeks or 6 months. But you can get excellent results.

There are also "free living studies" where participants live freely at home and you give them a certain diet plan or counseling to get them to do what you want. These are less well controlled, but they can be done fairly accurately in some cases.

Then you have prospective studies where you give participants a plan to follow and check in with them frequently to see how they are doing and if they are sticking to the plan.

There are studies called Meta Analysis where they look at multiple studies and multiple data sets and try to draw conclusions from aggregating data.

There are all kinds of diet research studies that can be done. Some are better than others, but the point is, you have to evaluate all of these and come up with conclusions that are generalizable and actionable. Not all study methodologies are equal. Sometimes you can find very well done free living studies, and sometimes you can find poorly done metabolic ward studies. The point is, you have to look at the totality of evidence and come up with meaningful conclusions and takeaways. Watch my 1.5 hour "Diet Research Review" on YouTube (DrAlo.tv).

Another factor you have to take into consideration is human behavior. Sure, we can recommend a low carb diet for all to follow, but how likely is it that humans will actually follow this long term? Studies have shown that people who try to follow a low carb diet can only adhere to it for a few months. They start out eating less than 30g of carbs per day, but after a year they are eating 100g of carbs or more, but when questioned, they still think they are eating a low carb diet. Human behavior is complicated and not always easy to assess. You must adapt your strategies to human behavior.

Diet vs Exercise?

When I am lecturing on weight loss, I always survey the audience, "What's more important, diet or exercise?"

About 30% raise their hand for diet, about 40% for exercise, and the rest try to say both or don't raise their hands at all.

Weight loss is all diet! That's right. You can not outrun a bad diet. And you can't outlift one either, if you are into weightlifting. It's just not possible. Sure, the two can work together, but the majority of weight loss comes from diet alone.

Recent studies have shown that the more you exercise, the more your body will reduce your metabolic rate. Your body can lower your metabolism by 28% if needed, and if you are obese, you can have a 50% reduction in metabolism. So exercise can be a double edged sword. More on this later.

The exercise part can help you look different in the end, once you have adjusted your diet and lost weight. If you lifted heavy weights while dieting, you will look nicer and more toned. If you ran or did cardio, you will look very lean, but could also end up skinny fat. We will get into this more later.

Diet Exercise

In case you need a visual, look up! Weight loss is 97% diet!

Multiple studies have been done on this and you can watch my 1.5 hour lecture on YouTube (DrAlo.tv) for an in depth review of all relevant exercise studies. Search for my "Exercise Research Review".

The Journal of the American Medical Association published one such study. Here are the results in graphic format from the study. You can watch that video if you want more exercise research.

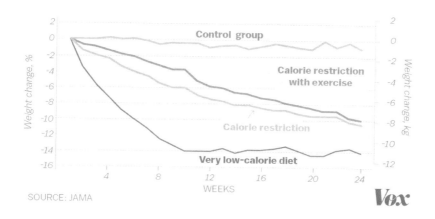

SOURCE: JAMA

45

As you can see from the above chart, the group that did "Diet Only" lost more weight than the group that did diet and exercise. This is due to many different reasons. Firstly, in some people diet increases appetite. Another reason, is that some people may eat more if they exercise thinking it's ok to eat more since they are exercising, i.e. human behavior. Other reasons are the body's multitude of adaptation mechanisms. We dive deeper into these topics later.

Take a look at the study below. Adding exercise or "depending on exercise" to cause the majority of your weight loss, will not work. So many studies have been done on this. I will post some below and highlight the conclusions, you can go through them on your own.

Effects of aerobic versus resistance exercise without caloric restriction on abdominal fat, intrahepatic lipid, and insulin sensitivity in obese adolescent boys: a randomized, controlled trial. Diabetes, 61(11), 2787-2795
Lee, S., Bacha, F., Hannon, T., Kuk, J. L., Boesch, C., & Arslanian, S. (2012).

A 3-month randomized, controlled study **[4]** recruited 43 overweight or obese adolescent boys (12-18 years old) who were physically inactive which was quantified as no participation in structured physical activity over the previous 3 months except school physical education classes. All subjects were asked to follow a weight maintenance diet during the 3-month intervention period to determine the effects of exercise without caloric restriction. Subjects were split into three groups: aerobic exercise, resistance training, or control. The aerobic exercise program consisted of treadmill, elliptical, or stationary bike sessions three times per week for 60 minutes per session at approximately 50% of VO2peak and increased to 60 minutes at 60-75% of VO2peak by week two. The resistance training program consisted of ten exercises such as leg press, chest press, latissimus pull downs, seated row, among others. The week 1-4 protocol was to perform 1-2 sets of 8-12 repetitions at 60% of baseline. During weeks 4-12, subjects performed two sets of 8-12 repetitions to fatigue.

While these are not the most challenging training protocols known to mankind, keep in mind that these are adolescent boys who have puberty to thank for the plethora of androgenic hormones pumping through their veins for the first time and they are also novice exercisers which will allow them to make faster progress than any other population. These two factors, adolescent in age and novice exercisers, should create a perfect cocktail where exercise could make a huge impact on body composition.

However, the data showed that after three months, exercise had very little impact on weight loss. (Remember, 1 lb.= 2.2 kgs.)

- Control group gained 2.6 + 1.0 kg body weight
- Aerobic exercise group lost 0.04 + 0.8 kg body weight
- Resistance training group lost 0.6 + 0.8 kg body weight

Obes Rev. 2009 May;10(3):313-23. doi: 10.1111/j.1467-789X.2008.00547.x. Epub 2009 Jan 19.

Long-term effectiveness of diet-plus-exercise interventions vs. diet-only interventions for weight loss: a meta-analysis.

Wu T[1], Gao X, Chen M, van Dam RM.

+ Author information

Abstract

Diet and exercise are two of the commonest strategies to reduce weight. Whether a diet-plus-exercise intervention is more effective for weight loss than a diet-only intervention in the long-term has not been conclusively established. The objective of this study was to systemically review the effect of diet-plus-exercise interventions vs. diet-only interventions on both long-term and short-term weight loss. Studies were retrieved by searching MEDLINE and Cochrane Library (1966 - June 2008). Studies were included if they were randomized controlled trials comparing the effect of diet-plus-exercise interventions vs. diet-only interventions on weight loss for a minimum of 6 months among obese or overweight adults. Eighteen studies met our inclusion criteria. Data were independently extracted by two investigators using a standardized protocol. We found that the overall standardized mean differences between diet-plus-exercise interventions and diet-only interventions at the end of follow-up were -0.25 (95% confidence interval [CI]-0.36 to -0.14), with a P-value for heterogeneity of 0.4. Because there were two outcome measurements: weight (kg) and body mass index (kg m(-2)), we also stratified the results by weight and body mass index outcome. The pooled weight loss was 1.14 kg (95% CI 0.21 to 2.07) or 0.50 kg m(-2) (95% CI 0.21 to 0.79) greater for the diet-plus-exercise group than the diet-only group. We did not detect significant heterogeneity in either stratum. Even in studies lasting 2 years or longer, diet-plus-exercise interventions provided significantly greater weight loss than diet-only interventions. In summary, a combined diet-plus-exercise programme provided greater long-term weight loss than a diet-only programme. However, both diet-only and diet-plus-exercise programmes are associated with partial weight regain, and future studies should explore better strategies to limit weight regain and achieve greater long-term weight loss.

PMID: 19175510 [PubMed - indexed for MEDLINE]

Even in the studies that showed that exercise plus diet worked, it was a 0.5 to 1.14Kg weight loss over 2 years. That's 1-2 pounds at the most.

Total Daily Energy Expenditure (TDEE)

It's important to define some terms before we begin. Total daily energy expenditure is made up of several components.

Component of TDEE	% of TDEE (approximate)	Definition	Change during Weight Loss
Basal Metabolic Rate (BMR)	70%	Amount of energy required to keep bodily functions processing at rest	Weight loss reduces metabolically active tissue which decreases BMR
Non-Exercise Activity Thermogenesis (NEAT)	15%	Energy expended during "non-exercise" movement such as fidgeting or normal daily activities	Evidence suggests that NEAT is decreased when in caloric restriction and remain reduced even after subjects return to freely feeding
Thermic Effect of Food (TEF)	10%	Energy expended during process of ingesting, absorbing, metabolizing, and storing nutrients from food	Magnitude maintains but overall reduction because of caloric restriction
Exercise Activity Thermogenesis (EAT)	5%	Energy used during exercise	Exercise will increase this component but as you continue exercising with a weight loss goal, a reduction in body mass will reduce the energy requirement needed to complete a given amount of activity. Meaning as you lose weight, you expend less energy for the same amount of activity.

Modified from Trexler, Smith-Ryan, & Norton, 2014 [8] Trexler, E. T., Smith-Ryan, A. E., & Norton, L. E. (2014). Metabolic adaptation to weight loss: implications for the athlete. Journal of the International Society of Sports Nutrition, 11(1). 7.

The first one is basic metabolic rate (BMR). This is about 70% of your total daily energy expenditure. This is the amount of energy you need to "keep the lights on" if your body is fully at rest. This is the bare minimum amount of calories you need to stay alive if you stayed in bed all day and didn't move.

The next biggest component is non exercise activity thermogenesis (NEAT). This comprises about 15% of your total daily energy expenditure. This is all your imperceptible movements. This is your fidgeting, moving, shifting, walking, talking with your hands, and the amount of steps you do daily. This is not purposeful exercise.

Next is the thermic effect of food (TEF). This comprises about 10% of your total daily energy expenditure. This is the amount of energy it takes your body to breakdown and utilize the food that you have eaten.

Last is exercise activity thermogenesis (EAT). This comprises about 5% of your total daily energy expenditure. This is purposeful exercise activity. This is you going to the gym. This is you riding a bike. This is purposeful exercise. This is when you "workout". Notice, it's just 5%.

As you can see, exercise does not play a major role in your total daily energy expenditure. It's very difficult to exercise enough to surpass that 5% threshold. And in fact, if you do exercise more, you won't necessarily burn more calories. That's why it's much more effective to focus on total caloric intake, i.e. your diet, than worrying about walking or exercising away your calories. As you'll see next, exercising more does not necessarily equal more calories burned.

Constrained Model of Exercise

One thing we've also learned is that exercise is not linear. Exercise is not endless in the amount of calories that it can burn. Studies have shown that you cannot simply just do more exercise to burn more calories and therefore increase your total of daily energy expenditure. We now believe in a constrained model of physical activity. That you can exercise up to a certain point and you will burn more up to a certain point. But you can not burn more calories beyond a certain point.

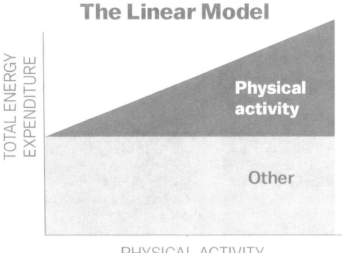

The Linear Model

TOTAL ENERGY EXPENDITURE

Physical activity

Other

PHYSICAL ACTIVITY

SOURCE: Current Biology (2016)

This is the previously believed linear model of physical activity. We used to believe that the more you exercise, the more calories you burn. This is no longer true.

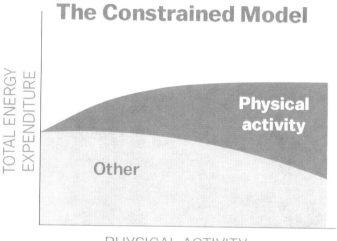

The Constrained Model

TOTAL ENERGY EXPENDITURE

Physical activity

Other

PHYSICAL ACTIVITY

SOURCE: Current Biology (2016)

We now know that there is a cap to the amount of calories you can burn with exercise. When you first start exercising you will burn more calories up to a certain point, then you no longer burn more calories. In fact, your body will downregulate other parts of your total daily energy expenditure to make up and compensate for it. This usually comes from non exercise activity thermogenesis (NEAT). You will stop fidgeting, stop moving, stop walking as much, and stop doing other imperceptible movements that you didn't even know you had.

Here's the study if you want to look at it and of course you can watch my very in-depth exercise YouTube video. Go to DrAlo.tv and search for "In Depth Exercise Research Review".

Constrained Total Energy Expenditure and Metabolic Adaptation to Physical Activity in Adult Humans

Herman Pontzer, Ramon Duran, Andou, Lara R. Dugas, Richard S. Cooper, Dale A. Schoeller, Amy Luke
https://doi.org/10.1016/j.cub.2015.12.046

Highlights

- We measured total energy expenditure and physical activity in a large adult sample
- Above moderate activity levels, total energy expenditure plateaued
- Body fat percentage was positively related to total energy expenditure
- Activity intensity was inversely related to total energy expenditure

Summary

Current obesity prevention strategies recommend increasing daily physical activity, assuming that increased activity will lead to corresponding increases in total energy expenditure and prevent or reverse energy imbalance and weight gain [1, 2, 3]. Such Additive total energy expenditure models are supported by exercise intervention and accelerometry studies reporting positive correlations between physical activity and total energy expenditure [4] but are challenged by ecological studies in humans and other species showing that more active populations do not have higher total energy expenditure [5, 6, 7, 8]. Here we tested a Constrained total energy expenditure model, in which total energy expenditure increases with physical activity at low activity levels but plateaus at higher activity levels as the body adapts to maintain total energy expenditure within a narrow range. We compared total energy expenditure, measured using doubly labeled water, against physical activity, measured using accelerometry, for a large (n = 332) sample of adults living in five populations [9]. After adjusting for body size and composition, total energy expenditure was positively correlated with physical activity, but the relationship was markedly stronger over the lower range of physical activity. For subjects in the upper range of physical activity, total energy expenditure plateaued, supporting a Constrained total energy expenditure model. Body fat percentage and activity intensity appear to modulate the metabolic response to physical activity. Models of energy balance employed in public health [1, 2, 3] should be revised to better reflect the constrained nature of total energy expenditure and the complex effects of physical activity on metabolic physiology.

A similar study showed the same results and can be accessed at: https://pubmed.ncbi.nlm.nih.gov/25906426/

Below are the findings and graphic from that study.

Report

Current Biology

Energy compensation and adiposity in humans

Highlights

- Energy compensation in humans was analyzed from daily and basal energy expenditure
- Reduced BEE results in energy compensation of 28%
- Degree of energy compensation varied between people of different body composition

Authors

Vincent Careau, Lewis G. Halsey, Herman Pontzer, ..., William W. Wong, Yosuke Yamada, John R. Speakman

Correspondence

vcareau@uottawa.ca (V.C.),
l.halsey@roehampton.ac.uk (L.G.H.),
herman.pontzer@duke.edu (H.P.),
aluke@luc.edu (A.H.L.),
jennifer.rood@pbrc.edu (J.R.),
sagayama.hiroyuki.ka@u.tsukuba.ac.jp (H.S.),
dschoell@nutrisci.wisc.edu (D.A.S.),
wwong@bcm.edu (W.W.W.),
yyamada831@gmail.com (Y.Y.),
j.speakman@abdn.ac.uk (J.R.S.)

In brief

Energy compensation is the concept that not all the energy spent when activity levels increase translates to additional energy spent that day, but it is poorly characterized. Careau, Halsey et al. find that in humans, energy compensation averages 28%, i.e., only 72% of the extra calories we spend on additional activity translates into extra calories burned that day.

SUMMARY

Understanding the impacts of activity on energy balance is crucial. Increasing levels of activity may bring diminishing returns in energy expenditure because of compensatory responses in non-activity energy expenditures.[1-3] This suggestion has profound implications for both the evolution of metabolism and human health. It implies that a long-term increase in activity does not directly translate into an increase in total energy expenditure (TEE) because other components of TEE may decrease in response—energy compensation. We used the largest dataset compiled on adult TEE and basal energy expenditure (BEE) (n = 1,754) of people living normal lives to find that energy compensation by a typical human averages 28% due to reduced BEE; this suggests that only 72% of the extra calories we burn from additional activity translates into extra calories burned that day. Moreover, the degree of energy compensation varied considerably between people of different body compositions. This association between compensation and adiposity could be due to among-individual differences in compensation: people who compensate more may be more likely to accumulate body fat. Alternatively, the process might occur within individuals: as we get fatter, our body might compensate more strongly for the calories burned during activity, making losing fat progressively more difficult. Determining the causality of the relationship between energy compensation and adiposity will be key to improving public health strategies regarding obesity.

The study demonstrated that when you exercise, your body compensates by reducing your BMR by up to 28%. People who were more overweight, had more adaptation and compensation. This shows that the more overweight you are, the harder it may be to burn more calories with more exercise.

Below are some of the graphics from the study.

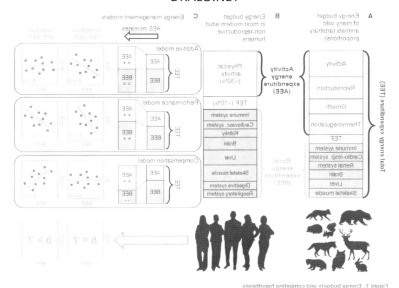

It's a very complicated subject and new data is suggesting that more exercise does not necessarily result in more calories burned. You are welcome to click the links above and look at the diagrams and explanations for a more detailed review.

Exercise Wrap Up

There are obviously many benefits to exercise. We know that exercise lowers your blood pressure, lowers your cholesterol, lowers insulin resistance, and improves overall mortality and cardiovascular mortality. We also know that exercise is very good at keeping you from gaining weight back that you've already lost. If you enjoy exercise, you should do what you enjoy. Pick an activity that you like and just keep doing it for fun. But do not depend on exercise for weight loss. We must learn how to create a calorie deficit with food alone. We will get into creating a calorie deficit later. Your body is pretty good at adapting to most forms of exercise.

Exercise:

- The amount of exercise you'd have to do to lose weight is time prohibitive.
- Burning an extra 500 calories per day would require jogging for 5-6 miles per day.
- That may take 90-120 minutes.
- The amount of energy you can burn from physical activity is capped and constrained.
- Exercise is good for keeping lost weight off, but will not help you lose excessive weight
- Eating less and healthier is the key
- Exercise suppresses and or increases appetite
- Exercise activates fight/flight response and puts the rest/digest system on hold
- Exercise lowers cardiovascular mortality significantly (which is huge!)
- Exercise alone inefficient for weight loss
- Lowers BP, LDL, blood sugar
- Increase HDL
- Prevents weight re-gain
- Increase/Decrease hunger
- Activates compensatory adaptive mechanisms
- Does not cause significant weight loss

And I want to stress this once again, exercise is excellent at reducing cardiovascular mortality. Just take a look at the study below from the Journal of the American College of Cardiology from 2014. They found that walking at a very slow pace, even just two to three mph, just one or two times per week, decreases cardiovascular mortality by 45%. If you were to do that every day it would reduce cardiovascular mortality by 50%. And they found that this reduces all-cause mortality by 29%. All-cause mortality means that the chance of you getting hit by a bus and dying is also reduced by 29%.

Mortality

J Am Coll Cardiol. 2014;64(5):472-481

- Running at even at a slow pace for 5-10 minutes just 1 or 2 times per week decreases cardiovascular mortality by 45%
- Doing it every day reduces cardiovascular mortality by 50%
- Reduced all cause mortality by 29%

Please don't go tell your friends that the cardiologist said not to do cardio! I always joke at all my lectures that I'm a "cardio" ologist! Cardio is part of my name. It's very good for you, it's just not the best and most sustainable way to lose weight. There's a much better way, which is why I wrote this book!

Human behavior plays a huge role in this. Can you run every day for the rest of your life? Into your 80s and 90s? Can you lift weights 6 days a week forever? Can you swim every day for the rest of your life? Sure, all of those things can burn calories. Just not as much as we'd like. And your body can adapt to that and constrain calorie burn and energy expenditure. So we have to find a way to create a calorie deficit without depending on exercise. So that you can do it for a very long time. Yes, we can do things like diet breaks and go on maintenance phases to bring our metabolism back up. But we don't want to be overly reliant on exercise for creating a calorie deficit.

You should do activities that you enjoy and maintain a certain level of activity. If your fitness tracker says you are doing 5000 steps a day, try to get to 8500 and set that as your minimum. Don't go crazy running and jogging and trying to torture yourself into losing weight.

If 5000 is all you got, then that's fine. Set your calorie deficit up and stick to at least 5000 steps.

Make sure you do things you enjoy and aren't punishing yourself with exercise. If you like to golf, then do that. If you like to walk, then do that. By the way, walking is one of those activities that they body's adaptive mechanisms can't adapt to, so you can do that daily. But still try not to depend on hundreds of miles a week of walking to create your calorie deficit.

Chapter 4

Appetite Regulation, Perception, and Control

Another big problem, is appetite regulation is off if you are overweight. Studies have found that the more overweight you are, and the less active you are, the more your appetite is dysregulated. Meaning, you are not aware of how much food you really have to eat. So, your body may be signaling to you that you are still hungry, when you are actually quite full.

Here is a landmark study showing this effect. Again you can go through the details with me in my in-depth exercise research review video, which will be linked at the end of this book. But take a look below.

Homeostatic and non-homeostatic appetite control along the spectrum of physical activity levels: An updated perspective

Kristine Beaulieu [1], Mark Hopkins [2], John Blundell [3], Graham Finlayson [3]
Affiliations
•PMID: 29289613
•DOI: 10.1016/j.physbeh.2017.12.032
Free article

Abstract

The current obesogenic environment promotes physical inactivity and food consumption in excess of energy requirements, two important modifiable risk factors influencing energy balance. Habitual physical activity has been shown to impact not only energy expenditure, but also energy intake through mechanisms of appetite control. This review summarizes recent theory and evidence underpinning the role of physical activity in the homeostatic and non-homeostatic mechanisms controlling appetite. Energy intake along the spectrum of physical activity levels (inactive to highly active) appears to be J-shaped, with low levels of physical activity leading to dysregulated appetite and a mismatch between energy intake and expenditure. At higher levels, habitual physical activity influences homeostatic appetite control in a dual-process action by increasing the drive to eat through greater energy expenditure, but also by enhancing post-meal satiety, allowing energy intake to better match energy expenditure in response to hunger and satiety signals. There is clear presumptive evidence that physical activity energy expenditure can act as a drive (determinant) of energy intake. The influence of physical activity level on non-homeostatic appetite control is less clear, but low levels of physical activity may amplify hedonic states and behavioural traits favouring overconsumption indirectly through increased body fat. More evidence is required to understand the interaction between physical activity, appetite control and diet composition on passive overconsumption and energy balance. Furthermore, potential moderators of appetite control along the spectrum of physical activity, such as body composition, sex, and type, intensity and timing of physical activity, remain to be fully understood.

Key Points

1. Physical activity does more than just increase total energy expenditure. When activity is low, appetite is dysregulated, resulting in excess food intake and weight gain. Higher levels of activity seem to increase appetite control.
2. The combination of being too high in body fat and also being physically inactive may further dysregulate appetite and satiety signaling, making weight loss efforts even more difficult.
3. Physical activity and exercise may only be effective to a point for the goal of weight loss. At very high levels of physical activity, additional increases may not result in an increase in total energy expenditure, but rather a downregulation of energy expended from other components of total energy expenditure and no change in net expenditure.

It's not Your Metabolism

A point that must be made now is that it's not your metabolism. Many of my friends, patients, and clients tell me that they can't lose weight because their metabolism has slowed down. I used to give them examples of so many older patients and friends that have lost weight successfully, even after age 40, 50, 60, and even 70. But now we have studies that show that your metabolism does not slow down.

A recent study in Science showed that daily energy expenditure (metabolism) does not decrease between ages 20 and 60. Yes, your metabolism is higher if you are 5-10 years old, and still quite high up until about age 20. But then levels off until you reach age 60. It was a very well-done study using doubly labelled water with a very varied population, including tons of women at multiple stages of pregnancy. And their metabolism was no different either.

Take a look at the graph below for a visual representation of metabolism over the years.

A

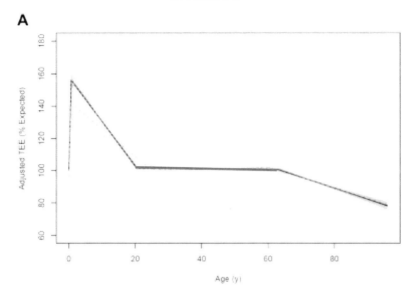

Here's the study for those who need more!

Science

REPORT   METABOLISM

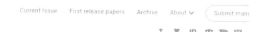

Daily energy expenditure through the human life course

HERMAN PONTZER   YOSUKE YAMADA   HIROYUKI SAGAYAMA   PHILIP N. AINSLIE LENE F. ANDERSEN   LIAM J. ANDERSON LENORE ARAB

ISSAD BADDOU   KWEKU BEDU-ADDO   IAEA DLW DATABASE CONSORTIUM   +74 authors   Authors Info & Affiliations

SCIENCE · 13 Aug 2021 · Vol 373, Issue 6556 · pp. 808-812 · DOI: 10.1126/science.abe5017

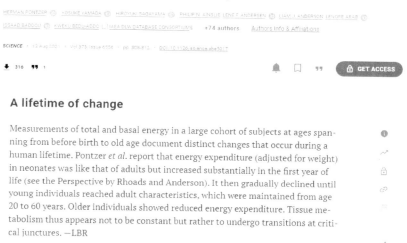

GET ACCESS

A lifetime of change

Measurements of total and basal energy in a large cohort of subjects at ages spanning from before birth to old age document distinct changes that occur during a human lifetime. Pontzer *et al.* report that energy expenditure (adjusted for weight) in neonates was like that of adults but increased substantially in the first year of life (see the Perspective by Rhoads and Anderson). It then gradually declined until young individuals reached adult characteristics, which were maintained from age 20 to 60 years. Older individuals showed reduced energy expenditure. Tissue metabolism thus appears not to be constant but rather to undergo transitions at critical junctures. —LBR

Abstract

Total daily energy expenditure ("total expenditure") reflects daily energy needs and is a critical variable in human health and physiology, but its trajectory over the life course is poorly studied. We analyzed a large, diverse database of total expenditure measured by the doubly labeled water method for males and females aged 8 days to 95 years. Total expenditure increased with fat-free mass in a power-law manner, with four distinct life stages. Fat-free mass–adjusted expenditure accelerates rapidly in neonates to ~50% above adult values at ~1 year; declines slowly to adult levels by ~20 years; remains stable in adulthood (20 to 60 years), even during pregnancy; then declines in older adults. These changes shed light on human development and aging and should help shape nutrition and health strategies across the life span.

You can access the study at:
https://www.science.org/doi/abs/10.1126/science.abe5017

Why Do People Lose Weight When They Start Exercising?

My friend and his wife started running last year during the pandemic. They were mostly sedentary, but decided that running was a safe outdoor activity that shouldn't spread covid. They both lost 10-15 pounds in the first 2 months. Great. A few months later, they were back to their starting weight, if not higher. So why is that?

Studies have shown that when someone starts any new exercise program (any new activity, like running, biking, walking, lifting weights, etc) they will lose a small amount of weight in the first few months. Only to gain it back later.

Physical activity, total and regional obesity: dose-response considerations

R Ross †, I Janssen
Affiliations
•PMID: 11427779
•DOI: 10.1097/00005768-200106001-00023

Abstract

Purpose: This review was undertaken to determine whether exercise-induced weight loss was associated with corresponding reductions in total, abdominal, and visceral fat in a dose-response manner.

Methods: A literature search (MEDLINE, 1966--2000) was performed using appropriate keywords to identify studies that consider the influence of exercise-induced weight loss on total and/or abdominal fat. The reference lists of those studies identified were cross-referenced for additional studies.

Results: Total fat. Review of available evidence suggested that studies evaluating the utility of physical activity as a means of obesity reduction could be subdivided into two categories based on study duration. Short-term studies (< or = 16 wk, N = 20) were characterized by exercise programs that increased energy expenditure by values double (2200 vs 1100 kcal.wk-1) that of long-term studies (> or = 26 wk, N = 11). Accordingly, short-term studies report reductions in body weight (-0.18 vs -0.06 kg x wk(-1)) and total fat (-0.21 vs -0.06 kg x wk(-1)) that are threefold higher than those reported in long-term studies. Moreover, with respect to dose-response issues, the evidence from short-term studies suggest that exercise-induced weight loss is positively related to reductions in total fat in a dose-response manner. No such relationship was observed when the results from long-term studies were examined. Abdominal fat. Limited evidence suggests that exercise-induced weight loss is associated with reductions in abdominal obesity as measured by waist circumference or imaging methods; however, at present there is insufficient evidence to determine a dose-response relationship between physical activity, and abdominal or visceral fat.

Conclusion: In response to well-controlled, short-term trials, increasing physical activity expressed as energy expended per week is positively related to reductions in total adiposity in a dose-response manner. Although physical activity is associated with reduction in abdominal and visceral fat, there is insufficient evidence to determine a dose-response relationship.

And there are many other studies like this. This shows a dose response. When you first start an exercise program, you will lose weight for about 3 months. Then you have to work really hard, or really control calories to maintain that weight loss, because of your body's adaptive mechanisms. The short-term studies showed weight loss (not much though) but all of the longer-term studies showed no weight loss from exercise.

Another study compared weight loss from diet alone versus weight loss from diet with aerobic training.

Ann Nutr Metab. 2007;51(5):428-32. Epub 2007 Nov 20.

Fat loss depends on energy deficit only, independently of the method for weight loss.

Strasser B[1], Spreitzer A, Haber P.

⊞ Author information

Abstract

BACKGROUND: This study was designed to compare the effects of 2 different but isocaloric fat reduction programs with the same amount of energy deficit - diet alone or diet combined with aerobic training - on body composition, lipid profile and cardiorespiratory fitness in non- or moderately obese women.

METHODS: Twenty non- or moderately obese (BMI 24.32 +/- 3.11) females (27.3 +/- 6.6 years) were tested at the beginning and after an 8-week period of a mild hypocaloric diet for the following parameters: (1) body mass and body fat, (2) total cholesterol, HDL-C, LDL-C and triglycerides, (3) lactate (mmol/liter) during submaximal exertion (100 W), (4) heart rate during submaximal exertion (100 W), and (5) maximum exercise performance (watt). Subjects were randomly divided into either a diet alone (D, -2,095 +/- 659 kJ/day) or a diet (-1,420 +/- 1,084 kJ/day) plus exercise (DE, three 60-min sessions per week at 60% of VO(2)max or -5,866 kJ/week) group.

RESULTS: Body mass and body fat decreased significantly in D (-1.95 +/- 1.13 kg or -1.47 +/- 0.87%, p < 0.05) and DE (-2.23 +/- 1.28 kg or -1.59 +/- 0.87%, p < 0.05), but there was no significant difference observed between the groups. Statistical analysis revealed no significant changes of total cholesterol, HDL-C, LDL-C, triglycerides and heart rate during submaximal exertion (100 W). Lactic acid accumulation during submaximal exertion (100 W) decreased significantly (-0.8 +/- 1.4 mmol/l, p < 0.05) in DE and increased significantly (+0.4 +/- 0.5 mmol/l, p < 0.05) in D. Maximum exercise performance improved significantly (+12.2 +/- 8.8 W, p < 0.05) in DE and did not change significantly in D.

CONCLUSIONS: This study showed that independently of the method for weight loss, the negative energy balance alone is responsible for weight reduction.

The conclusion was that the negative energy balance *alone* was responsible for weight loss. The exercise had no effect. Only the calorie deficit mattered. Nothing else. No amount of exercise helped. Although, there is a type of exercise that can help with weight loss, we will discuss that later.

Muscle Matters

Yes, building muscle is going to matter. Sure, you can lose weight without gaining muscle but it's much better to lose weight while gaining muscle, or at least retaining as much muscle as possible. The more muscle you have the more protected you are against cancer, chronic illnesses, and cardiovascular mortality. Multiple studies have proven this and you can watch my full in depth exercise research review on <u>YouTube</u>.

More Muscle:
- Protects against cardiovascular mortality
- Protects against cancer
- Protects against chronic illness

History of Diets

Unfortunately, the United States government and the USDA have not had a good record when it comes to diets. They have tried very hard and they have done a good job with some things, but over the years the public has lost trust in them. Some of the lost trust is because some people selling diet books try to flip the food pyramids upside down claiming that their way is better. Unfortunately, this is not true. People who follow the keto diet or Atkins diet try to claim that the well-balanced diet that the USDA and government promotes is not as healthy or as good as a keto style diet which is heavy in meats and fats.

So, what do we make of this? First, we must take a look at the history of the USDA recommended diets.

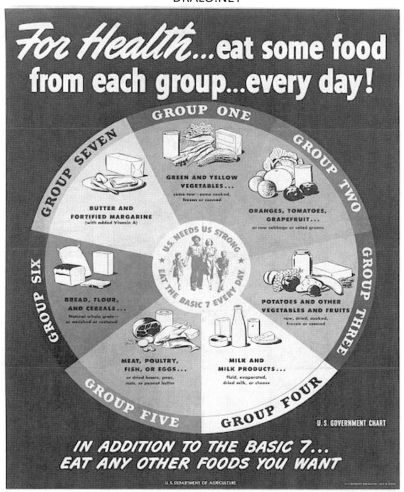

This was the USDA recommendation in 1943. They grouped everything into seven groups and created a pie chart with the various food groups in it. It was a good starting point for that time. But they wanted to make sure that all Americans ate at least something from these food groups so that they don't have vitamin deficiencies.

In 1992 the US government published the food pyramid which you can take a look at below that was heavy on whole grains at the bottom part of the pyramid. This is about the same time that the

Atkins and low carb diets became popular, hence they talked negatively about the USDA recommended diet.

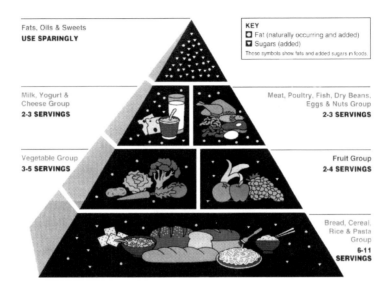

As you can see from above, it is very heavy on whole grains and carbohydrates, includes plenty of fruits and vegetables, but very small amounts of protein, and small amounts of dairy and fat. While this is an okay start, it's definitely not the most optimal diet for someone trying to lose weight and get fit and build muscle. It's a good place to start and we can refine this and get into the details later. The biggest issue with this is the lack of protein. You will need much more than the picture suggests.

In 2005 they wanted to fix this pyramid and emphasize physical activity hence they added a staircase to the side with a human running up the stairs to emphasize physical activity and stress that physical activity is also important.

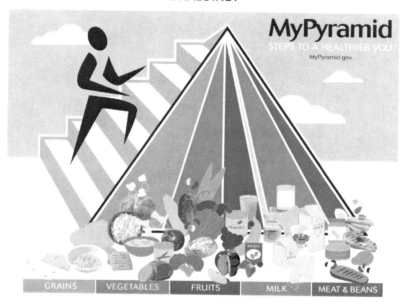

This was definitely an improvement, but you also notice that protein and dairy are not given much emphasis. There are plenty of fruits and vegetables mixed in, but milk gets its own category that is rather large (considering that dairy has a high amount of saturated fat). Emphasizing physical activity was important at the time and it was good that they did that, but as you'll see, physical activity alone and even in combination with diet, is not going to cause as much weight loss as diet alone, even without physical activity. A really good diet will be all that you need.

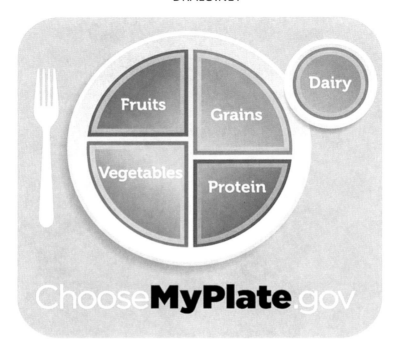

In 2010, this was revised again, and this is probably the closest thing we have to what we probably should be eating, although I wouldn't emphasize dairy as much. In this version, they are using dairy in a cup to the side mainly to represent fats.

As you can see, there have been multiple iterations of this. Some of which have been pretty close to good, but still missed the mark. We will get into what makes the perfect diet for you, and it's not always the same for everyone. A lot of it depends on your goals. If you are looking to gain weight and bulk up, you are going to be eating much differently than someone who is looking to maintain their weight. If you are looking to lose weight, then there are certain macro nutrients that are non-negotiables that you have to eat enough of to minimize muscle loss and prevent lowering your basic metabolic rate.

Chapter 5

Introduction to Nutrition

Now that we know that nutrition is 97% of weight loss, let's get started! Once again, you can't outrun or out exercise or out lift your diet. There's really no point in even discussing exercise if your nutrition isn't fixed first.

Step One: Fix your nutrition and eating
Step Two: Adopt an exercise program that meets your goals

You need to develop a nutrition plan that includes all the foods that you like, so that you can stick to it long term. More on that later.

I want you to develop a healthy relationship with food and exercise.

I want you to lose weight while eating foods that you like!

Calories

A calorie is the amount of energy it takes to raise the temperature of one gram of water by 1 degree Celsius. The amount of calories in food is measured in a calorimeter. They take that food and burn it inside of a sealed container and they see how much the temperature of water changes. But for most of us, we really don't need to know any of that.

When it comes to food, calories are reported with a capital C which is actually kilocalories. So, when you see 1 Calorie, it's actually 1000 kcal. But for the sake of simplicity, we won't go into detail and just use the term calories.

Calories listed on food labels, are total calories. Calories matter the most when it comes to weight loss. There are some nuances, but if you wanted to just lose weight, you need to eat less calories than you take in. Obviously, this isn't going to work if you are already eating only 1200 calories a day and are still overweight. So, you will need to know what to do in that scenario, which we will discuss later. There are a lot of people in this exact dilemma. This is called metabolic adaptation and there are ways to get out of it.

One gram of carbohydrates is 4 calories. Same for protein. But one gram of fat is 9 calories. Fat is more energy dense. Alcohol is in between, at around 7 calories per gram.

These numbers don't matter all that much other than to just give you an idea of how much a gram of the various foods is "worth".

Macros

Macronutrients are the larger components of food. The carbohydrates, proteins, and fats. Micronutrients are the microscopic components of food, like vitamins, minerals, cholesterol, iron, magnesium, etc.

Sure, you can lose weight by ignoring macronutrition, but you may not like how you look at the end. It won't be optimal. You may end up skinny fat and can lose muscle in the process. That's why we stress getting your protein and macros right.

This section discusses macronutrients and how they can contribute to proper weight loss. How can you use macronutrition to optimize your weight loss and look your best!

Protein

Protein is the main macronutrient that we focus on in our weight loss discussions because it is crucial to losing fat and not losing muscle. You need to eat enough protein to maintain your muscle or even gain muscle. If you are a woman, don't worry, you aren't going to get bulky and big. More on that later.

Protein is found in most meat products; beef, chicken, fish, turkey, eggs, pork, etc. The meat of these animals contains protein. But other foods can too; chick peas, lentils, peas, beans, nuts, eggs, yogurt, quinoa, and others.

You can use whey protein powders to supplement your intake if you aren't getting enough. The biggest problem is when you are trying to get enough protein by eating normal foods and you end up going over your calories. One way to avoid this is by eating whey protein shakes to avoid going over your calories, but still get enough protein.

If you are vegetarian, you can use vegetable protein powders to supplement your intake. In the section in the back there is a vegetarian protein guide.

Protein is the only macronutrient that you have to actually consume, because there are certain proteins called "essential amino acids" that your body needs and can't produce on it's own.

Fats

Fats are important, but no essential! They are important for hormone synthesis. Hormones that cause muscle growth and retention, like testosterone. Women need these for their hormones as well. It's hard to lose weight when your fat levels go too low, and you can't make the right hormones. The good news is, that your body can still synthesize hormones if needed, even if you aren't eating fat.

Fats are not absolutely essential! You don't have to actually eat any fat, and your body can still make them. Keep that in mind.

This is why, after setting up protein goals, we set up fat goals. You want to make sure you are getting enough fat that your body can still make sufficient hormones.

Fats are more calorie dense compared to carbohydrates and proteins. Fats are 9 calories per gram of fat, while protein and carbs are 4 calories per gram.

Something like a ribeye steak or bacon, contains a good amount of protein, but the fat content can increase its total caloric burden or "cost". You need to be conscious of these decisions and choices.

Carbs

Carbohydrates are the "sugars" or main fuel source. They can be divided into processed and unprocessed. They can also be categorized as simple or complex.

A simple sugar (processed carb) can be absorbed pretty quickly. Most of the digestion has already been done for you. Imagine taking an apple and blending it up into a smoothie. You've already started the breakdown process and it's easier for your stomach to access the sugars. But if you bite into a whole apple, it's harder to gain access to the sugars because of all of the fiber surrounding them.

We set your carbs up last (after protein and fat) because they can be any number and can vary heavily from person to person. Whatever remaining calories you have left can be carbs.

This will fuel your workouts later.

Can you cut out carbs? Sure, it's the only macronutrient that you can technically reduce severely and still be ok. But not optimal for long term adherence and to fuel your body and workouts.

Chapter 6

What if I Want to Eat Low Carb?

I have a lot of people tell me they are on Keto or Atkins style diets eating low carbs and that they are losing weight doing that. Sure, that can work for some people, but only if calories are restricted. Plenty of people gain weight eating "low carb" but eating 5000 calories per day.

So many studies have now been done where they kept calories the same (isocaloric) and varied the amount of carbs the participants ate to see if there was a difference in weight loss. And there is no difference. Even better, some studies controlled protein as well. See below for one of the better studies on this.

A randomized trial comparing low-fat and low-carbohydrate diets matched for energy and protein

C J Segal-Isaacson [1], Shannah Johnson, Vlad Tomuta, Brandy Cowell, Daniel T Stein

Affiliations
•PMID: 15601961
•DOI: 10.1038/oby.2004.278

Abstract

Several recent studies have found greater weight loss at 6 months among participants on a very-low-carbohydrate (VLC) weight-loss diet compared with a low-fat (LF) weight-loss diet. Because most of these studies were not matched for calories, it is not clear whether these results are caused by decreased energy intake or increased energy expenditure. It is hypothesized that several energy-consuming metabolic pathways are up-regulated during a VLC diet, leading to increased energy expenditure. The focus of this study was to investigate whether, when protein and energy are held constant, there is a significant difference in fat and weight loss when fat and carbohydrate are dramatically varied in the diet. The preliminary results presented in this paper are for the first four of six postmenopausal overweight or obese participants who followed, in random order, both a VLC and an LF diet for 6 weeks. Other outcome measures were serum lipids, glucose, and insulin, as well as dietary compliance and side effects. Our results showed no significant weight loss, lipid, serum insulin, or glucose differences between the two diets. Lipids were dramatically reduced on both diets, with a trend for greater triglyceride reduction on the VLC diet. Glucose levels were also reduced on both diets, with a trend for insulin reduction on the VLC diet. Compliance was excellent with both diets, and side effects were mild, although participants reported more food cravings and bad breath on the VLC diet and more burping and flatulence on the LF diet.

https://pubmed.ncbi.nlm.nih.gov/15601961/

If you keep calories and protein the same, it makes no difference if you eat a very low carb or low fat diet, you will still lose the same amount of weight.

The above study was very well done and answered that exact question. When you compare two isocaloric diets, meaning they are both the same amount of calories, you will lose the same amount of weight, regardless of the macronutrient breakdown of those diets. It does not matter if you eat 90% fat or 90% carbs or 90% protein, you still lose the same amount of weight. They have tested all different combinations and ratios of macronutrients and the results are always the same. If you match calories and protein and vary everything else, it doesn't matter, you still lose the same amount of weight. (More studies in the appendix in the back)

What about Low Glycemic Index Foods versus High Glycemic Index Foods

I have a lot of patients and friends that tell me they switched to eating more complex carbs than simple carbs, hoping that this will cause weight loss. And it can, if you end up eating higher volume foods that are lower calorie. For example, you could eat three cucumbers and that's like 23 calories. It will fill you up. It's mostly fiber and complex carbs. If you ate this instead of eating a Pop Tart, then sure, it will help you because you are eating less total calories. A Pop Tart will take up less space in your stomach, but is about 250 calories.

But lets say you are eating 250 calories of Doritos vs 250 of zucchini. Sure, the Doritos will spike your blood sugar more (high glycemic index), while the zucchini will not (low glycemic index). But the overall caloric burden is the same. There's no difference when it comes to weight loss. You can lose weight eating high or low glycemic index foods, as long as you control total calories and get enough protein.

This has been studied extensively and we know the answers. Take a look at the studies below. (More studies in the appendix in the back)

No effect of a diet with a reduced glycaemic index on satiety, energy intake and body weight in overweight and obese women

L M Aston [1], C S Stokes, S A Jebb

Affiliations
•PMID: 17923862
•PMCID: PMC2699494
•DOI: 10.1038/sj.ijo.0803717
Free PMC article

Abstract

Objective: To investigate whether a diet with a reduced glycaemic index (GI) has effects on appetite, energy intake, body weight and composition in overweight and obese female subjects.

Design: Randomized crossover intervention study including two consecutive 12-week periods. Lower or higher GI versions of key carbohydrate-rich foods (breads, breakfast cereals, rice and pasta/potatoes) were provided to subjects to be incorporated into habitual diets in ad libitum quantities. Foods intended as equivalents to each other were balanced in macronutrient composition, fibre content and energy density.
Subjects: Nineteen overweight and obese women, weight-stable, with moderate hyperinsulinaemia (age: 34-65 years, body mass index: 25-47 kg m(-2), fasting insulin: 49-156 pmol l(-1)).

Measurements: Dietary intake, body weight and composition after each 12-week intervention. Subjectively rated appetite and short-term ad libitum energy intake at a snack and lunch meal following fixed lower and higher GI test breakfasts (GI 52 vs 64) in a laboratory setting.

Results: Free-living diets differed in GI by 8.4 units (55.5 vs 63.9), with key foods providing 48% of carbohydrate intake during both periods. There were no differences in energy intake, body weight or body composition between treatments. On laboratory investigation days, there were no differences in subjective ratings of hunger or fullness, or in energy intake at the snack or lunch meal.

Conclusion: This study provides no evidence to support an effect of a reduced GI diet on satiety, energy intake or body weight in overweight/obese women. Claims that the GI of the diet per se may have specific effects on body weight may therefore be misleading.

Ketogenic low-carbohydrate diets have no metabolic advantage over nonketogenic low-carbohydrate diets

Carol S Johnston [1], Sherrie L Tjonn, Pamela D Swan, Andrea White, Heather Hutchins, Barry Sears

•PMID: 16685046
•DOI: 10.1093/ajcn/83.5.1055

Background: Low-carbohydrate diets may promote greater weight loss than does the conventional low-fat, high-carbohydrate diet.

Objective: We compared weight loss and biomarker change in adults adhering to a ketogenic low-carbohydrate (KLC) diet or a nonketogenic low-carbohydrate (NLC) diet.

Design: Twenty adults [body mass index (in kg/m(2)): 34.4 +/- 1.0] were randomly assigned to the KLC (60% of energy as fat, beginning with approximately 5% of energy as carbohydrate) or NLC (30% of energy as fat; approximately 40% of energy as carbohydrate) diet. During the 6-wk trial, participants were sedentary, and 24-h intakes were strictly controlled.

Results: Mean (+/-SE) weight losses (6.3 +/- 0.6 and 7.2 +/- 0.8 kg in KLC and NLC dieters, respectively; P = 0.324) and fat losses (3.4 and 5.5 kg in KLC and NLC dieters, respectively; P = 0.111) did not differ significantly by group after 6 wk. Blood beta-hydroxybutyrate in the KLC dieters was 3.6 times that in the NLC dieters at week 2 (P = 0.018), and LDL cholesterol was directly correlated with blood beta-hydroxybutyrate (r = 0.297, P = 0.025). Overall, insulin sensitivity and resting energy expenditure increased and serum gamma-glutamyltransferase concentrations decreased in both diet groups during the 6-wk trial (P < 0.05). However, inflammatory risk (arachidonic acid:eicosapentaenoic acid ratios in plasma phospholipids) and perceptions of vigor were more adversely affected by the KLC than by the NLC diet.

Conclusions: KLC and NLC diets were equally effective in reducing body weight and insulin resistance, but the KLC diet was associated with several adverse metabolic and emotional effects. The use of ketogenic diets for weight loss is not warranted.

No significant difference in weight loss or insulin resistance. Low fat keto caused several adverse metabolic and emotional effects.

What About Eating an Anti-Inflammatory Diet?

There are a lot of people selling books and diets that are "anti-inflammatory". Guess what? There's really no such thing as a diet that is inflammatory. If you are losing weight, you are reducing inflammation. There is nothing more inflammatory than being obese. Fat cells (adipocytes) are very pro inflammatory and are always releasing pro inflammatory markers. Take a look at the studies below.

Published in final edited form as:
Int J Cardiol. 2020 January 15; 299: 282–288. doi:10.1016/j.ijcard.2019.07.102.

Healthy diet reduces markers of cardiac injury and inflammation regardless of macronutrients: results from the OmniHeart trial

Lara C. Kovell, MD[1], Edwina H. Yeung, PhD[2], Edgar R. Miller III, MD, PhD[3], Lawrence J. Appel, MD, MPH[4], Robert H. Christenson, PhD[5], Heather Rebuck, MS[6], Steven P. Schulman, MD[7], Stephen P. Juraschek, MD, PhD[8]

[1]Division of Cardiology, University of Massachusetts Medical School, Worcester, MA. This author takes responsibility for all aspects of the reliability and freedom from bias of the data presented and their discussion interpretation;

Abstract

Background: Despite diet being a first-line strategy for preventing cardiovascular disease, the optimal macronutrient profile remains unclear. We studied the effects of macronutrient profile on subclinical cardiovascular injury and inflammation.

Methods: OmniHeart was a randomized 3-period, crossover feeding study in 164 adults with high blood pressure or hypertension (SBP 120-159 or DBP 80-99 mm Hg). Participants were fed each of 3 diets (emphasizing carbohydrate (CARB), protein (PROT), or unsaturated fat (UNSAT)) for 6-weeks, with feeding periods separated by a washout period. Weight was held constant. Fasting serum was collected at baseline while participants ate their own diets and after each feeding period. High-sensitivity troponin I (hs-cTnI) and high-sensitivity C-reactive protein (hs-CRP) were measured in stored specimens.

Results: The average age was 53.6 years, 55% were African American, and 45% were women. At baseline, the median (25th-percentile, 75th-percentile) hs-cTnI was 3.3 ng/L (1.9, 5.6) and hs-CRP was 2.2 mg/L (1.1, 5.2). Compared to baseline, all 3 diets reduced hs-cTnI: CARB −8.6% (95%CI: −16.1, −0.4), PROT −10.8% (−18.4, −2.5), and UNSAT −9.4% (−17.4, −0.5). Hs-CRP was similarly changed by −13.9 to −17.0%. Hs-cTnI and hs-CRP reductions were of similar magnitudes as SBP and low-density lipoprotein cholesterol (LDLc) but were not associated with these risk-factor reductions (*P-values*=0.09). There were no between-diet differences in hs-cTnI and hs-CRP reductions.

Conclusions: Healthy diet, regardless of macronutrient emphasis, directly mitigated subclinical cardiac injury and inflammation in a population at risk for cardiovascular disease. These findings support dietary recommendations emphasizing healthy foods rather than any one macronutrient.

Just read that conclusion.

Regardless of which macronutrients you decide to emphasize, you will lower inflammation if you are in a calorie deficit and weight is coming off.

Isocaloric Diets High in Animal or Plant Protein Reduce Liver Fat and Inflammation in Individuals With Type 2 Diabetes

Mariya Markova [2], Olga Pivovarova [2], Silke Hornemann [2], Stephanie Sucher [2], Turid Frahnow [3], Katrin Wegner [4], Jürgen Machann [5], Klaus Jürgen Petzke [6], Johannes Hierholzer [7], Ralf Lichtinghagen [8], Christian Herder [9], Maren Carstensen-Kirberg [9], Michael Roden [9], Natalia Rudovich [10], Susanne Klaus [6], Ralph Thomann [11], Rosemarie Schneeweiss [12], Sascha Rohn [13], Andreas F H Pfeiffer [1].
Affiliations

•PMID: 27765690
•DOI: 10.1053/j.gastro.2016.10.007

Abstract

Background & aims: Nonalcoholic fatty liver disease (NAFLD) is associated with increased risk of hepatic, cardiovascular, and metabolic diseases. High-protein diets, rich in methionine and branched chain amino acids (BCAAs), apparently reduce liver fat, but can induce insulin resistance. We investigated the effects of diets high in animal protein (AP) vs plant protein (PP), which differ in levels of methionine and BCAAs, in patients with type 2 diabetes and NAFLD. We examined levels of liver fat, lipogenic indices, markers of inflammation, serum levels of fibroblast growth factor 21 (FGF21), and activation of signaling pathways in adipose tissue.

Methods: We performed a prospective study of individuals with type 2 diabetes and NAFLD at a tertiary medical center in Germany from June 2013 through March 2015. We analyzed data from 37 subjects placed on a diet high in AP (rich in meat and dairy foods; n = 18) or PP (mainly legume protein; n = 19) without calorie restriction for 6 weeks. The diets were isocaloric with the same macronutrient composition (30% protein, 40% carbohydrates, and 30% fat). Participants were examined at the start of the study and after the 6-week diet period for body mass index, body composition, hip circumference, resting energy expenditure, and respiratory quotient. Body fat and intrahepatic fat were detected by magnetic resonance imaging and spectroscopy, respectively. Levels of glucose, insulin, liver enzymes, and inflammation markers, as well as individual free fatty acids and free amino acids, were measured in collected blood samples. Hyperinsulinemic euglycemic clamps were performed to determine whole-body insulin sensitivity. Subcutaneous adipose tissue samples were collected and analyzed for gene expression patterns and phosphorylation of signaling proteins.

Results: Postprandial levels of BCAAs and methionine were significantly higher in subjects on the AP vs the PP diet. The AP and PP diets each reduced liver fat by 36%-48% within 6 weeks (for AP diet P = .0002; for PP diet P = .001). These reductions were unrelated to change in body weight, but correlated with down-regulation of lipolysis and lipogenic indices. Serum level of FGF21 decreased by 50% in each group (for AP diet P < .0002; for PP diet P < .0002); decrease in FGF21 correlated with loss of hepatic fat. In gene expression analyses of adipose tissue, expression of the FGF21 receptor cofactor β-klotho was associated with reduced expression of genes encoding lipolytic and lipogenic proteins. In patients on each diet, levels of hepatic enzymes and markers of inflammation decreased, insulin sensitivity increased, and serum level of keratin 18 decreased.

Conclusions: In a prospective study of patients with type 2 diabetes, we found diets high in protein (either animal or plant) significantly reduced liver fat independently of body weight, and reduced markers of insulin resistance and hepatic necroinflammation. The diets appear to mediate these changes via lipolytic and lipogenic pathways in adipose tissue. Negative effects of BCAA or methionine were not detectable. FGF21 level appears to be a marker of metabolic improvement. ClinicalTrials.gov ID NCT02402985.

Keywords: FFA; KLB; NAFLD; NASH.

If you want to read more on inflammation, here's a few more links:

Inflammation not different between ketogenic diet and low fat diet when calories are equated:
https://pubmed.ncbi.nlm.nih.gov/12949361/

Omega 3 PUFAs may decrease inflammation:
https://journals.lww.com/md-journal/Fulltext/2017/02170/Impact_of_the_dietary_fatty_acid_intake_on.6.aspx

Sugar intake does not increase inflammation in absence of weight gain:
https://academic.oup.com/ajcn/article/82/2/421/4862989?login=true

In looking at the totality of the research available, there's really no such thing as a pro-inflammatory diet, other than just consuming too many calories. Cut back your calories and your inflammation will come down with weight loss.

Now, I am not that dogmatic and stringent. If there are certain foods that you don't like, or cause you bloating, or give you diarrhea, acne, and belching, then obviously avoid those. But don't let anyone sell you anything that sounds like and "anti-inflammatory" diet because somehow it is superior to all other forms of weight loss. Just like the prior example with Intermittent Fasting. Yes, it can work for you, but it is not the **only** way to lose weight. Run if anyone is telling you things like that.

The same goes for a ketogenic style diet, if it fits into your lifestyle and you enjoy those foods, and CAN MAINTAIN IT LONG TERM, then go for it. But human behavior studies have shown that most people can't maintain this style of eating long term.

If you are a cardiac patient and have had a heart attack or stroke or have high cholesterol with other risk factors, you should not be doing a keto style diet. At least not one with high levels of saturated fat. You can select healthier fats. More on saturated fats and red meat below.

What About Intermittent Fasting?

A lot of people like to do intermittent fasting to help with weight loss. In the scientific literature we call this Intermittent Energy Restriction (IER). Multiple studies have looked at Intermittent Energy Restriction vs a Continuous Energy Restriction (eating in a calorie deficit daily without regard to timing, or not eating for entire days) and have no difference in weight loss, cardiovascular risk factors, LDL, blood pressure, and insulin resistance. All improved. Here's one recent Metanalysis that was just published in 2021. A Metanalysis is a review of multiple studies. Unfortunately, too many intermittent fasting studies don't control for calories, it's nice to find studies that are well done and control for calories.

Meta-Analysis > Crit Rev Food Sci Nutr. 2021;61(8):1293-1304.
doi: 10.1080/10408398.2020.1757616. Epub 2020 May 2.

Impact of intermittent energy restriction on anthropometric outcomes and intermediate disease markers in patients with overweight and obesity: systematic review and meta-analyses

Lukas Schwingshackl [1], Jasmin Zähringer [1], Kai Nitschke [1], Gabriel Torbahn [2], Szimonetta Lohner [3], Tilman Kühn [4], Luigi Fontana [5] [6], Nicola Veronese [7], Christine Schmucker [1], Joerg J Meerpohl [1] [8]

Affiliations + expand

PMID: 32363896   DOI: 10.1080/10408398.2020.1757616

Abstract

This systematic review aims to investigate the effects of intermittent energy restriction (IER) on anthropometric outcomes and intermediate disease markers. A systematic literature search was conducted in three electronic databases. Randomized controlled trials (RCTs) were included if the intervention lasted ≥12 weeks and IER was compared with either continuous energy restriction (CER) or a usual diet. Random-effects meta-analysis was performed for eight outcomes. Certainty of evidence was assessed using GRADE. Seventeen RCTs with 1328 participants were included. IER in comparison to a usual diet may reduce body weight (mean difference [MD]: -4.83 kg, 95%-CI: -5.46, -4.21; n = 6 RCTs), waist circumference (MD: -1.73 cm, 95%-CI: -3.69, 0.24; n = 2), fat mass (MD: -2.54 kg, 95%-CI: -3.78, -1.31; n = 6), triacylglycerols (MD: -0.20 mmol/L, 95%-CI: -0.38, -0.03; n = 5) and systolic blood pressure (MD: -6.11 mmHg, 95%-CI: -9.59, -2.64; n = 5). No effects were observed for LDL-cholesterol, fasting glucose, and glycosylated-hemoglobin. Both, IER and CER have similar effect on body weight (MD: -0.55 kg, 95%-CI: -1.01, -0.09; n = 13), and fat mass (MD: -0.66 kg, 95%-CI: -1.14, -0.19; n = 10), and all other outcomes. In conclusion, IER improves anthropometric outcomes and intermediate disease markers when compared to a usual diet. The effects of IER on weight loss are similar to weight loss achieved by CER.

https://pubmed.ncbi.nlm.nih.gov/32363896/

There was no difference in weight loss. There was however, more lean body mass loss in the IER group. This is a pattern we have seen in intermittent fasting studies

Another study from 2021 also looked at IER versus CER and also found no difference weight loss or other health markers. This study compared the 5:2 method of fasting, where you let participants eat whatever they want for 5 days, then have them fast for 2 days.

The point I am trying to make is that intermittent fasting can work for you if it fits into your preferences and schedule. Some people have a busy morning and don't care to eat and don't feel hungry until about 1pm anyways, so this may work for them. I am not against that. Please go ahead and use this strategy. But I am against people that say that this is the only way to lose weight.

https://pubmed.ncbi.nlm.nih.gov/34733895/

> Front Cardiovasc Med. 2021 Oct 18;8:750714. doi: 10.3389/fcvm.2021.750714. eCollection 2021.

Effects of Intermittent Compared With Continuous Energy Restriction on Blood Pressure Control in Overweight and Obese Patients With Hypertension

Chao-Jie He [1], Ye-Ping Fei [1], Chun-Yan Zhu [2], Ming Yao [2], Gang Qian [1], Hui-Lin Hu [1], Chang-Lin Zhai [1]

Affiliations + expand
PMID: 34733895   PMCID: PMC8558476   DOI: 10.3389/fcvm.2021.750714
Free PMC article

Abstract

Background and Aims: Weight-loss diets reduce body weight and improve blood pressure control in hypertensive patients. Intermittent energy restriction (IER) is an alternative to continuous energy restriction (CER) for weight reduction. We aimed to compare the effects of IER with those of CER on blood pressure control and weight loss in overweight and obese patients with hypertension during a 6-month period. **Methods:** Two hundred and five overweight or obese participants (BMI 28.7 kg/m^2) with hypertension were randomized to IER (5:2 diet, a very-low-calorie diet for 2 days per week, 500 kcal/day for women and 600 kcal/day for men, along with 5 days of a habitual diet) compared to a moderate CER diet (1,000 kcal/day for women and 1,200 kcal/day for men) for 6 months. The primary outcomes of this study were changes in blood pressure and weight, and the secondary outcomes were changes in body composition, glycosylated hemoglobin A1c (HbA1c), and blood lipids. **Results:** Of the 205 randomized participants (118 women and 87 men; mean [SD] age, 50.2 [8.9] years; mean [SD] body mass index. 28.7 [2.6]; mean [SD] systolic blood pressure, 143 [10] mmHg; and mean [SD] diastolic blood pressure, 91 [9] mmHg), 173 completed the study. The intention-to-treat analysis demonstrated that IER and CER are equally effective for weight loss and blood pressure control: the mean (SEM) weight change with IER was -7.0 [0.6] kg vs. -6.8 [0.6] kg with CER, the mean (SEM) systolic blood pressure with IER was -7 [0.7] mmHg vs. -7 [0.6] mmHg with CER, and the mean (SEM) diastolic blood pressure with IER was -6 [0.5] mmHg vs. -5 [0.5] mmHg with CER, (diet by time P = 0.62, 0.39, and 0.41, respectively). There were favorable improvements in body composition, HbA1c, and blood lipid levels, with no differences between groups. Effects did not differ according to completer analysis. No severe hypoglycemia occurred in either group during the trial. **Conclusions:** Intermittent energy restriction is an effective alternative diet strategy for weight loss and blood pressure control and is comparable to CER in overweight and obese patients with hypertension. **Clinical Trial Registration:** http://www.chictr.org.cn, identifier: ChiCTR2000040468.

Another issue is that intermittent fasting has been shown to reduce lean body mass (muscle mass). We want to avoid losing muscle mass. However, intermittent fasting (or any calorie restriction) combined with resistance training can help mitigate muscle loss and accelerate fat loss. It's very important to strength traing while in a calorie deficit. More on this later.

What About Artificial Sweeteners and the Gut Microbiome?

The gut microbiome is the collection of bacteria that sit inside your intestines and help break down food products for use. Studies say that we have more bacterial cells in our intestines than human cells in our body.

You see a lot of online influencers talk about artificial sweeteners and having bad effects on your gut microbiome. Of course, they are usually selling some type of supplement or plan that is supposed to improve your gut microbiome. The research is very clear that artificial sweeteners do not affect your gut microbiome. At all. Not one bit.

Take a look at this very well done study below.

Randomized Controlled Trial   > Nutrients. 2020 Nov 6;12(11):3409. doi: 10.3390/nu12113408

The Effects of Non-Nutritive Artificial Sweeteners, Aspartame and Sucralose, on the Gut Microbiome in Healthy Adults: Secondary Outcomes of a Randomized Double-Blinded Crossover Clinical Trial

Samar Y Ahmad [1], James Friel [1], Dylan Mackay [1,2]

Affiliations + expand

PMID: 33171964   PMCID: PMC7694690   DOI: 10.3390/nu12113408
Free PMC article

Abstract

Non-nutritive artificial sweeteners (NNSs) may have the ability to change the gut microbiota, which could potentially alter glucose metabolism. This study aimed to determine the effect of sucralose and aspartame consumption on gut microbiota composition using realistic doses of NNSs. Seventeen healthy participants between the ages of 18 and 45 years who had a body mass index (BMI) of 20-25 were selected. They undertook two 14-day treatment periods separated by a four-week washout period. The sweeteners consumed by each participant consisted of a standardized dose of 14% (0.425 g) of the acceptable daily intake (ADI) for aspartame and 20% (0.136 g) of the ADI for sucralose. Faecal samples collected before and after treatments were analysed for microbiome and short-chain fatty acids (SCFAs). There were no differences in the median relative proportions of the most abundant bacterial taxa (family and genus) before and after treatments with both NNSs. The microbiota community structure also did not show any obvious differences. There were no differences in faecal SCFAs following the consumption of the NNSs. These findings suggest that daily repeated consumption of pure aspartame or sucralose in doses reflective of typical high consumption have minimal effect on gut microbiota composition or SCFA production.

https://pubmed.ncbi.nlm.nih.gov/33171964/

Can your gut microbiome be influenced by what you eat? Yes, it can. If you eat more fat, you will overproduce bacteria like *A. muciniphila* and *Lactobacillus* to help break down the fat better. Your microbiome can adapt to what you eat. We are learning more and more about the gut microbiome and how it can modulate certain chronic disease states and help us fight off certain disease or improve our response to certain disease. The research is ongoing on this. If you want to learn more about the current state of gut microbiome research, take a look at this long study. It's a very nice overview of what we currently know about the gut microbiome and chronic illness and possible pathways that disease and the microbiome intersect.

Saturated Fat: The Debate Ends

So, what are saturated fats? These are fats that are solid at room temperature. These are foods like butter, bacon, lard, cheese, margarine, coconut oil, fat on steak, chicken skin, fat in ground beef, etc. These are the most atherogenic fats that cause the most plaque build up in your arteries. This is not a question. This is a fact. It's been established over and over again in science and literature. Any of these internet or Instagram gurus trying to tell you that saturated fat doesn't matter, are absolutely wrong and completely clueless. Can you eat some saturated fat? Sure, if you are pretty lean, like we described above.

In 1972, the North Karelia province in Finland had the highest cardiovascular mortality in the world. They had 700 deaths per 100,000. That was the highest in the world! The government decided to take a bunch of public health measures to help reduce mortality (death) in that region. They went in and taught everyone about heart disease, reduction in saturated fat intake, lower blood pressure, reduced smoking rates, and reducing obesity. People in North Karelia were rural and ate a lot of their calories from cheese, dairy, red meat, eggs, etc and were consuming upwards of 23% of their calories from saturated fat. They were able to lower it to below 12%, and even below 10%. They had an 84% reduction in mortality!

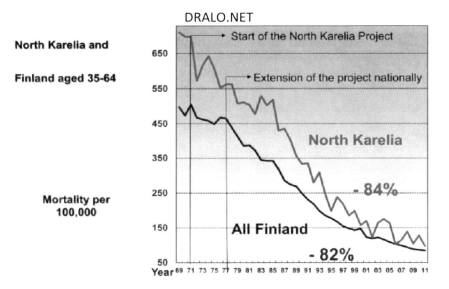

They weren't able to reduce smoking rates that much, in fact, smoking among women increased slightly, and obesity actually increased. Blood pressures did improve significantly. They attribute 40% of the reduction in mortality to the decrease in saturated fat intake and 20% to the reduction in blood pressure. Other factors did not play as significant a role.

Watch my video on YouTube discussing saturated fat.

Watch my YouTube video on 5 Things You Can Do To Live Longer. At about the 2:30 mark I discuss the Finland Study.

And here's the link to the full Article on North Karelia and Finland.

Saturated fats are also not "necessary". Your body can make what it needs. You don't have to consume x number of calories from saturated fat. Your hormones will still be in balance and your body can make what it needs. If you enjoy saturated fats, and who doesn't, like a nice ribeye every once in a while, try to keep saturated fat below 10% of total caloric intake.

Will Red Meat Kill You?

As a cardiologist I get asked this question all the time. "Hey doc, can I eat red meat?"

The answer is, it depends! Yeah, I know you didn't want to hear that. But if you are pretty lean and fit, you can get away with eating a little more red meat than people who are more overweight and especially when compared to obese individuals. If you are pretty lean and at a normal BMI, yes, you can eat a bit more red meat (saturated fat). But if your BMI (body mass index) is over 27 with one or more risk factors (hypertension, cholesterol, diabetes, male sex, prior heart attack or stroke, age over 45 for men, 55 for women), then you shouldn't allow red meat (saturated fat) to be more than 10% of total calories. If your BMI is over 30, keep your saturated fat intake below 10% of all calories.

The study below shows that whether participants ate a high fat diet or low fat, high protein diet, that they reduced cardiovascular mortality equally. Both groups were in a calorie deficit and lost the same amount of weight.

Long-term weight maintenance and cardiovascular risk factors are not different following weight loss on carbohydrate-restricted diets high in either monounsaturated fat or protein in obese hyperinsulinaemic men and women

Jennifer B Keogh-1, Natalie D Luscombe-Marsh, Manny Noakes, Gary A Wittert, Peter M Clifton

PMID: 17298712 DOI: 10.1017/S0007114507252687

The aim of this study was to determine after 52 weeks whether advice to follow a lower carbohydrate diet, either high in monounsaturated fat or low fat, high in protein had differential effects in a free-living community setting. Following weight loss on either a high monounsaturated fat, standard protein (HMF; 50 % fat, 20 % protein (67 g/d), 30 % carbohydrate) or a high protein, moderate (HP) (40 % protein (136 g/d), 30 % fat, 30 % carbohydrate) energy-restricted diet (6000 kJ/d) subjects were asked to maintain the same dietary pattern without intensive dietary counselling for the following 36 weeks. Overall weight loss was 6.2 (SD 7.3) kg (P < 0.01 for time with no diet effect, 7.6 (SD 8.1) kg, HMF v. 4.8 (SD 6.6) kg, HP). In a multivariate regression model predictors of weight loss at the end of the study were sex, age and reported percentage energy from protein (R2 0.22, P < 0.05 for the whole model). Fasting plasma insulin decreased (P < 0.01, with no difference between diets), 13.9 (SD 4.6) to 10.2 (SD 5.2) mIU/l, but fasting plasma glucose was not reduced. Neither total cholesterol nor LDL-cholesterol were different but HDL was higher, 1.19 (SD 0.26) v. 1.04 (SD 0.29) (P < 0.001 for time, no diet effect), while TAG was lower, 1.87 (SD 1.23) v. 2.22 (SD 1.15) mmol/l (P < 0.05 for time, no diet effect). C-reactive protein decreased (3.97 (SD 2.84) to 2.43 (SD 2.29) mg/l, P < 0.01). Food records showed that compliance to the prescribed dietary patterns was poor. After 1 year there remained a clinically significant weight loss and improvement in cardiovascular risk factors with no adverse effects of a high monounsaturated fat diet.

Essentially no difference in CV risk factors between the groups.

We conclude that the weight loss alone was responsible for the decrease in cardiovascular mortality, not the macronutrient composition of their diet.

As long as you are losing weight, your cardiovascular and all-cause mortality will be lower. I can't stress this enough.

Below is a study looking a red meat intake and cardiovascular risk biomarkers.

Effects of Total Red Meat Intake on Glycemic Control and Inflammatory Biomarkers: A Meta-Analysis of Randomized Controlled Trials

Lauren E O'Connor [1,2], Jung Eun Kim [2,3], Caroline M Clark [2], Wenbin Zhu [2], Wayne W Campbell [2]

•PMID: 32910818
• DOI: 10.1093/advances/nmaa096

Abstract
Our objective was to conduct a systematic review and meta-analysis to assess the effects of total red meat (TRM) intake on glycemic control and inflammatory biomarkers using randomized controlled trials of individuals free from cardiometabolic disease. We hypothesized that higher TRM intake would negatively influence glycemic control and inflammation based on positive correlations between TRM and diabetes. We found 24 eligible articles (median duration, 3 weeks) from 1172 articles searched in PubMed, Cochrane, and CINAHL up to August 2019 that included 1) diet periods differing in TRM; 2) participants aged ≥19 years; 3) included either men or women who were not pregnant/lactating; 4) no diagnosed cardiometabolic disease; and 5) data on fasting glucose, insulin, HOMA-IR, glycated hemoglobin (HbA1c), C-reactive protein (CRP), or cytokines. We used 1) a repeated-measures ANOVA to assess pre to post diet period changes; 2) random-effects meta-analyses to compare pre to post changes between diet periods with ≥ vs. <0.5 servings (35g)/day of TRM; and 3) meta-regressions for dose-response relationships. We grouped diet periods to explore heterogeneity sources, including risk of bias, using the National Heart, Lung, and Blood Institute's Quality Assessment of Controlled Interventions Studies. Glucose, insulin, and HOMA-IR values decreased, while HbA1c and CRP values did not change during TRM or alternative diet periods. There was no difference in change values between diet periods with ≥ vs. <0.5 servings/day of TRM [weighted mean differences (95% CIs): glucose, 0.040 mmol/L (-0.049, 0.129); insulin, -0.710 pmol/L (-6.582, 5.162), HOMA-IR, 0.110 (-0.072, 0.293); CRP, 2.424 nmol/L (-1.460, 6.309)] and no dose response relationships (P > 0.2). Risk of bias (85% of studies were fair to good) did not influence results. Total red meat consumption, for up to 16 weeks, does not affect changes in biomarkers of glycemic control or inflammation for adults free of, but at risk for, cardiometabolic disease. This trial was registered at PROSPERO as 2018 CRD42018096031.

A cohort study examined the relationship between relationship between red meat, BMI and inflammatory markers (CRP, TNF-α, and IL-6) in 1223 subjects. They did indeed find that red meat intake was associated with markers of inflammation. HOWEVER, when they corrected for the differences in BMI, the associations between red meat and inflammatory markers were no longer significant, while the associations between BMI and inflammation were.

Read the section in red. When they corrected for Body Mass Index, there was no additional risk from red meat intake. But if you are overweight and consumed more red meat, then you were in trouble.

The takeaway message is that being overweight and obese increases inflammation more than anything else. The best way to reduce cardiovascular risk and inflammation is to lower your body weight.

Having a Good Relationship With Food

One of the most important fundamentals I try to teach is to develop a good relationship with food. You must learn to treat food as a tool to accomplish your goals. If your goals currently are weight loss, you will need fewer calories, you need to get enough protein, and you need to eat things you enjoy so that you can do this for a very long time.

Learn to enjoy your food regardless of what it is. You don't have to view food as "bad" or "good". You can gain and lose weight eating any kind of food, even healthy food. Have you ever tried eating 5000 calories a day of salad and "healthy" food? You will certainly gain weight.

Almost all of the enjoyment you get from eating "bad" food will come from the first bite. So just enjoy one bite or a small serving and move on. Don't feel bad or guilty. Just enjoy your food and enjoy your life and move on.

Stay within your calorie limit and you will be fine long term.

Taking Diet Breaks

Research has shown that taking diet breaks helps with adherence. People get diet fatigue and need a mental and physical break from prolonged calorie deficits. It's hard and it's taxing. It can affect you mentally and physically. The MATADOR study showed that taking breaks from your diet and moving your calories up to maintenance (even if you gain a couple pounds initially) will give you better long-term results. It can also preserve muscle mass and you will look better in the end. Don't be afraid to raise your calories a bit and maintain for a few months before you go back at it. Long term results are also better and more sustainable. Take a look at the MATADOR study below.

Link to article:
https://pubmed.ncbi.nlm.nih.gov/28925405-intermittent-energy-restriction-improves-weight-loss-efficiency-in-obese-men-the-matador-study/?from_single_result=ijo2017206

Intermittent energy restriction improves weight loss efficiency in obese men: the MATADOR study

N.M Byrne [1], A.Sainsbury [1], N.A King [1], A.P Hills [1,2], R.E Wood [1,2]
Affiliations
•PMID: 28925405
•PMCID: PMC5803575
•DOI: 10.1038/ijo.2017.206
Free PMC article

Abstract

Background/objectives: The MATADOR (Minimising Adaptive Thermogenesis And Deactivating Obesity Rebound) study examined whether intermittent energy restriction (ER) improved weight loss efficiency compared with continuous ER and, if so, whether intermittent ER attenuated compensatory responses associated with ER.

Subjects/methods: Fifty-one men with obesity were randomised to 16 weeks of either: (1) continuous (CON), or (2) intermittent (INT) ER completed as 8 × 2-week blocks of ER alternating with 7 × 2-week blocks of energy balance (30 weeks total). Forty-seven participants completed a 4-week baseline phase and commenced the intervention (CON: N=23, 39.4±6.8 years, 111.1±9.1 kg, 34.3±3.0 kg m⁻; INT: N=24, 39.8±9.5 years, 110.2±13.8 kg, 34.1±4.0 kg m⁻). During ER, energy intake was equivalent to 67% of weight maintenance requirements in both groups. Body weight, fat mass (FM), fat-free mass (FFM) and resting energy expenditure (REE) were measured throughout the study.

Results: For the N=19 CON and N=17 INT who completed the intervention per protocol, weight loss was greater for INT (14.1±5.6 vs 9.1±2.9 kg; P<0.001). INT had greater FM loss (12.3±4.8 vs 8.0±4.2 kg; P<0.01), but FFM loss was similar (INT: 1.8±1.6 vs CON: 1.2±2.5 kg; P=0.4). Mean weight change during the 7 × 2-week INT energy balance blocks was minimal (0.0±0.3 kg). While reduction in absolute REE did not differ between groups (INT: -502±481 vs CON: -624±557 kJ d⁻; P=0.5), after adjusting for changes in body composition, it was significantly lower in INT (INT: -360±502 vs CON: -749±498 kJ d⁻; P<0.05).

Conclusions: Greater weight and fat loss was achieved with intermittent ER. Interrupting ER with energy balance 'rest periods' may reduce compensatory metabolic responses and, in turn, improve weight loss efficiency.

Key Points

- Despite the same energy deficit and the same total time spent in an energy deficit, a group taking two-week diet breaks after every two weeks of dieting lost ~50% more fat mass compared to a group dieting continuously for 16 weeks. However, due to the frequency of these breaks, the group performing diet breaks required 30 weeks to complete all 16 weeks of dieting.

- Additionally, resting energy expenditure dropped only half as much in the diet break group compared to the continuous diet group when adjusted for body composition. This may be why the difference in groups favored the diet break group to a greater degree after a six-month follow-up, indicating diet breaks may help with the maintenance of weight loss after a diet concludes.

- Diet breaks appear to reverse important physiological adaptations to an energy deficit, subsequently making the dieting period following a break more effective for fat loss. While increasing the time required to complete a diet as much as was done in this study is probably impractical, performing a diet break every 4-8 weeks versus every two weeks may be a useful strategy for physique competitors and weight class-restricted strength athletes to enhance fat loss and mitigate declines in resting energy expenditure.

They have found that taking a few weeks off from your diet can help with adherence and prevent more muscle loss. I normally recommend to patients and clients to diet for 3 months (calorie restriction) and then increase calories slightly back up to maintenance levels for two months. This also helps prevent metabolic adaptation. Metabolic adaptation is when the body adapts to your current lower level of calories by reducing your BMR and NEAT.

Chapter 7

Previous Diets

Most diets you have ever read about fall into one of the following categories:

- Portion control- Weight Watchers, Zone
- Prepared food- Nutrisystem, Jenny Craig
- Low Carb/High protein- Atkins, South Beach, Keto
- Liquid/Fad diets
- Mediterranean- most proven
- Raw- Paleo, Halleluiah, God, Caveman
- Vegetarian, Vegan, Plant Based
- Glycemic Index Diet
- Intermittent fasting
- Elimination diets (TB12, Whole30)

One thing that is important to point out is that **All Diets Work (for some time)!**

Yes, no matter what you start trying, you will see some initial results right away. That is well known. Just like when you start running or lifting weights, you will initially see a slight decrease in body weight. But then all the adaptive and compensatory mechanisms take over and you are back where you started.

Yes, there is research to support all of these diets. You can look up all the studies and you can find articles and research showing health benefits of every single diet. That's not the debate here. You can adopt any one of these styles of eating or plans if you want. Just make sure it's something you can adhere to long term. That's the key.

All these diets work by creating a calorie deficit. The First Law of Thermodynamics states that energy can not be created nor destroyed and must always be in balance. If you are eating more than you need, you will store the excess energy (calories) as fat (or build muscle if you are weight training in a calorie surplus). If you eat less, you will use energy from your fat stores (lose fat). You can not break this law, but you can find creative ways to trick yourself into eating less calories.

Let's take low carb diets as an example. Most Americans get 60-70% of their calories from carbohydrates. So, when you reduce your caloric intake by 60-70%, you are going to lose weight, and lose weight quickly (another no, no). It's not that the carbs were making you fat, it's that now you are eating 1200 calories per day, instead of 3600 calories per day (a 66% reduction). It's the calories. Not the actual macronutrient makeup of the calories.

The same thing goes for intermittent fasting. There's nothing magical about intermittent fasting. But if you restrict your eating window to eat 1pm to 4pm, you probably aren't going to be able to eat 4000 calories in those few hours. So naturally, you'll create a calorie deficit.

Here's a nice graphic that illustrates this concept.

How Named Diets Work for Weight Loss

Diet Name	Short Description	How it Works
Low Carb	Eat fewer carbs and more foods rich in protein and fats	By creating a caloric deficit
Ketogenic	Eat almost no carbs, some protein and mostly fats	By creating a caloric deficit
Low Fat	Avoid foods high in fats and eat mostly protein and carbs	By creating a caloric deficit
Intermittent Fasting	Restrict your eating period to only a few hours every day	By creating a caloric deficit
Weight Watchers	Points based system to help with portion control	By creating a caloric deficit
Paleo	Eat only minimally-processed "paleolithic" foods	By creating a caloric deficit

All these diets work by creating a calorie deficit. At least until you start compensating and eating more. Which is what I hope to address and fix so that you learn to lose weight and keep it off.

So What Is the Best Diet For You?

The best diet for you is the one you can adhere to the longest. Choose foods you enjoy, just limit the portion sizes and fit them into your calorie count. We will get into this later in the workshop section towards the end.

I like to stress eating foods that you enjoy. Eat foods that you've eaten for the last five to 10-20 years. There's no reason to significantly change your diet or eliminate certain foods, food groups, or macronutrients simply because you think you are on a diet and need to restrict the types of foods that you eat. You are way more likely to adhere to the diet if you eat the foods that you've always enjoyed. You just might have to eat a lot less of them. But you can still eat them. This is very, very important! Eat what you enjoy!

Check out the video I did on YouTube describing my fictitious patient "Leslie" and the best diet for Leslie. I'm not kidding, you have to go watch that video. It's required!

The Leslie Diet

Go to DrAlo.tv and search for The Leslie Diet

Welcome back!

My fictitious patient "Leslie" asked me, "What's the best diet?" My response was a quick, "It's called the Leslie Diet." You must eat what Leslie likes to eat. It must be things that you like. Things you always eat. It just has to be a lot less.

What about Meal Plans?

If you look up diets online or follow diet gurus on Instagram, they're always trying to sell you meal plans. Why? Because they can make money off of you, making you think that this is the only way to lose weight. Plus, they can keep selling you meal plans forever!

The problem with meal plans is that they are cookie cutter and not everyone may like the foods you put on the meal plans. Everyone likes different things, and if you send everyone the same meal plan, they will view it as a "diet" and temporary fix and gain all the weight back once the diet "ends".

I want you to change your life and eating forever, not just a few months. You have to view this as a 1-2 year plan. Maybe more in some cases. You didn't put on all that weight overnight; you can't take it off overnight either.

I am a huge proponent of eating foods that you like and enjoy and learning to eat within your calorie limit. It will take some getting used to, but it will work.

Chapter 8

Setting Up Your Macros and Calorie Deficit

There are so many online calculators for macros and so many different ways to calculate your calorie and macro goals.

The easiest way is to multiply your weight by 10. So, a 200 pound person needs to eat 2000 calories to lose weight. This is a great place to start. Try this for 3-4 weeks and adjust as needed. If weight is not coming off, lower it by 5-10% and try again. For women who are shorter than 5 foot 2 inches and weigh less than 160 pounds, you might have to start a little lower. But it's still ok to start here and adjust later.

You need 0.7 to 1.6 grams of protein per pound of body weight. So, a 200 pound person will need 140-180g of protein per day depending on their body fat percentage or how lean they are. Sure, you could eat more protein, but no one really needs more than 240g.

As a quick estimate, most men will likely need 120-180g protein per day. Most women will need 80-140g protein per day.

Most online calculators can help you with some numbers to at least get you started.

But this is the simplest way to do it.

Below is a screengrab from one of my online courses that will help you figure this out more visually and in a workbook format. If you want the full workbook and Weight Loss 101 Masterclass that goes with it, click on: https://dralo.net/weightloss

Calculations

DrAlo.net

Calorie Deficit

Your current weight: _____ X 10 = _____

Total Calories needed to lose weight: _____

Protein

Your lean body weight: _____ X 0.7 = _____

Your lean body weight: _____ X 1.6 = _____

Your protein needs are somewhere between these two numbers. Ideally you want to use your lean body mass, but you may not know that number. If you are 200 pounds and estimate your body fat percentage (based on pictures in next page) to be 25%, that means you are 150 pounds of lean body mass.

Fat

Your current weight: _____ X 0.3 = _____

This is a good place to start for daily fat intake

Carbs

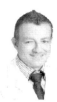

The rest of your calories can come from carbs

WEIGHT LOSS 101

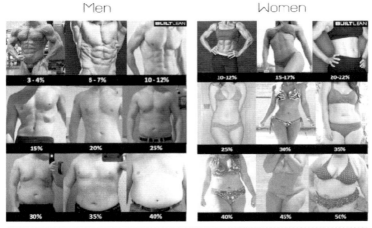

Use these pictures to estimate your body fat percentage for the previous page's calculations. For example, if you weigh 200 pounds and are 25% body fat, you would multiply 200 by 0.25 to get 50. So 50 pounds of your weight is fat and the other 150 is lean body mass. So your protein intake can be between 0.7 and 1.6 times 150. Usually, around 1g of protein per pound of lean body mass should be enough, so around 150g protein will work.

WEIGHT LOSS 101

The best way to track calories is using an app on your phone. They are super easy to use and make tracking super convenient. Don't worry, if you don't want to track calories or use an app, there's still a way to lose weight. You can skip to that section. But just read through this and give it a chance.

How to set up MyFitnessPal App

1. Don't pay for the premium version.

2. Register an account

3. Tell it your age, sex, height, current weight, and goal weight

4. Under the settings menu, go to Goals and adjust your Carbs/Protein/Fat to 40/40/20 ratio. This is a good place to start. Most men should end up with 120-180g of protein. Most women should end up with 80-140g protein. Try to get as close as possible.

5. Do not connect a fitness or step counter to the app. You want a calorie deficit with food alone, not through activity.

Using MyFitnessPal

Weigh yourself every morning wearing the same thing every day on a digital scale after you pee off your overnight pee. This is your lowest weight of the day. Just be consistent. Enter that weight every morning into the app.

Buy a digital food scale and weigh your food in grams and enter it. If you weigh a granny smith apple and it's 80g before you eat it, and the left-over core is 30g. Enter that you consumed 50g granny smith apple. This is the most accurate way to do it. Don't worry, you won't have to do this forever. You will eventually be able to look at food and know it's caloric value.

If a food has a barcode, use that. For example, white rice, scan the barcode, weigh it and tell the app you ate 100 grams of uncooked white rice, or if you cooked it, 180 grams cooked white rice.

Add your food before you eat it, so that you never overeat. Use the barcode scanner, it can really help.

Rule Number One

The number one rule is that you must hit your caloric goals! You don't want to be too far off in either direction. If you are too far below your goal, you will be hungry, lose weight too quickly, and never be able to maintain or sustain that type of diet long term. You will also lose a lot of muscle. If you are too far above your goal, you can end up staying at the same weight or even gaining weight if you string too many days together like that. Make sure your intake adds up to your calorie goal or is pretty close.

Rule Number Two

The second most important thing is to hit your protein goal every day. This will ensure that you retain as much muscle mass as possible and maybe even build muscle. This is for both men and women and does not change regardless of gender.

You will not have to track forever, but you need to learn about "what 1800 calories looks like". Eventually, you will know and can do it without tracking.

Don't worry if you are slightly off or just guessing. You just have to be close enough. We need to know that you are eating about 1800 calories a day and not 3000-4000. And it doesn't matter if your tracking isn't really accurate, we will adjust your calories based on the way that *you* track. So, if you track every green apple as just one medium green apple and you aren't losing weight, as we move on, we will lower your calories, and the way that you track will still work. It's a self-correcting mechanism. So don't worry too much about it.

What If You Don't Want to Count Calories

I have lots of patients that don't want to count calories. Yes, you can definitely lose weight without counting calories. It's a little trickier, but it can be done.

You have to think about your food and your plate visually. Cut everything in half and wait 20 minutes. If you are still hungry, go back and eat a little bit more. It takes 20 minutes for your stomach to realize that it's full and tell your brain that it's full. If you follow the simple plan of cutting all of your food in half visually and waiting 20 minutes, you will lose all the weight that you want. This way you will reduce your calories in half, and you should lose half your body weight. It's not as precise, but it's a good place to start if tracking scares you.

I explain this concept much better in this video. Go to DrAlo.tv and search for this:

<u>Losing Weight Without Counting Calories</u>

Welcome back!

Nutrition Timing Myths

For the vast majority of people, nutrition timing makes no difference. It doesn't matter if you eat most of your calories in two large meals or six small meals throughout the day, or one really big meal once a day. You are splitting hairs. If you are in a calorie deficit and eating the correct amount of calories, please just distribute them in a way that fits your schedule long term. We want to form lifelong habits and be able to fit this into your current lifestyle. We don't want to force you into waking up at 2am and 4am to get in a quick meal. That doesn't work long term. You will never do that for the next 50 years.

Does nutrition timing matter if you are a body builder? Sure. It does. You want to get some protein and carbs withing 30-90 minutes after your work out, and sometimes during your workout. But even then, you will probably be fine if you don't.

Just keep it simple and eat when it's convenient for you and don't overthink it.

Don't Fear Hunger!

You have to feel slightly hungry when you go to sleep at night. If you are full or feel stuffed, then you are not in a calorie deficit.

Don't be afraid to feel hungry! You need to be slightly hungry, that means you are in a calorie deficit. Embrace this and enjoy it.

Hunger is different than starvation. You don't want to feel like you are starving, just slightly hungry.

Obviously, if you are overweight your appetite regulation is not perfect and you may not actually feel hungry. This is why tracking calories is very important. We talked about appetite dysregulation previously. If you are overweight your body's appetite signaling may not be functioning properly.

Substitution

Substituting high-volume, low-calorie foods for lower volume, higher calorie foods is very important. You have to learn how to do this very, very well. If you are eating 1500 calories a day and have only 200 calories left at night, but you are still a little hungry, you could eat two cucumbers and feel pretty full and only have consumed 14 calories. You could also eat a bag of Doritos which is 300 calories but you don't feel full at all. Take advantage of foods that are very low calorie but take up a lot of space in your stomach. Any green vegetable, lots of water, carbonated zero calorie drinks and most raw vegetables fit this category. You can easily eat a salad of diced up onions, tomatoes, cucumbers, and lettuce with some Balsamic vinegar and salt and feel very full while consuming almost 0 calories.

Can You Gain Weight Eating Clean and Healthy?

Yes, you can lose weight while eating "bad" food.

Yes, you can gain weight eating "clean and healthy" food.

The composition of the food makes almost no difference when it comes to weight loss.

The head of nutrition at Kansas State University, Professor Mark Haubes, proved this while losing weight, eating only Twinkies. Watch my Twinkie Diet video and come back. Go to DrAlo.tv and search for: Twinkie Diet.

Welcome back!

Yes, he lost 28 pounds in ten weeks eating 100 grams of protein per day in a shake, which is only 400 calories, while the rest of his calories came from Twinkies, Little Debbie Cakes, Doritos, and Oreos. He ate 1800 calories a day of all junk food and lost 28 pounds in 10 weeks. He made sure to get protein because he didn't want to lose muscle, after all, he is the head of nutrition.

On top of all of that, his bad cholesterol (LDL) went down, his insulin resistance improved, his blood pressure improved, and all other measurable inflammatory markers improved, and his energy levels went up. All of the health benefits are conferred from the weight loss alone. Watch my 2 hour long in depth weight loss lecture for more on that. (DrAlo.tv)

So yes, you can lose weight eating foods that are less nutritious. But it's not as optimal. You will be hungrier as well because those foods are less filling

Healthiest Diet?

The Mediterranean diet is wholesome and nutritious and the only one with research studies showing that it reduces cardiovascular mortality, all-cause mortality, and many types of cancers.

You can still eat some foods that are not as wholesome and nutritious, but make sure 80% of your diet is wholesome and nutritious. This will help you with your weight loss goals and will make it easier to adhere to your diet.

But if you don't care and you like Twinkies and other junk food, yes, you can lose all the weight you want eating just that, as long as it adds up to your calorie limit.

Here's one of many studies showing benefits to a Mediterranean style diet.

BMC Med. 2014 Jul 24;12:112. doi: 10.1186/1741-7015-12-112

Definitions and potential health benefits of the Mediterranean diet: views from experts around the world.

Trichopoulou A[1], Martinez-Gonzalez MA, Tong TY, Forouhi NG, Khandelwal S, Prabhakaran D, Mozaffarian D, de Lorgeril M.

⊕ Author information

Abstract
The Mediterranean diet has been linked to a number of health benefits, including reduced mortality risk and lower incidence of cardiovascular disease. Definitions of the Mediterranean diet vary across some settings, and scores are increasingly being employed to define Mediterranean diet adherence in epidemiological studies. Some components of the Mediterranean diet overlap with other healthy dietary patterns, whereas other aspects are unique to the Mediterranean diet. In this forum article, we asked clinicians and researchers with an interest in the effect of diet on health to describe what constitutes a Mediterranean diet in different geographical settings, and how we can study the health benefits of this dietary pattern.

And another showing reduction in new cancers and overall mortality.

Curr Atheroscler Rep. 2013 Dec;15(12):370. doi: 10.1007/s11883-013-0370-4

Mediterranean diet and cardiovascular disease: historical perspective and latest evidence.

de Lorgeril M.

⊕ Author information

Abstract
The concept that the Mediterranean diet was associated with a lower incidence of cardiovascular disease (CVD) was first proposed in the 1950s. Since then, there have been randomized controlled trials and large epidemiological studies that reported associations with lower CVD: in 1994 and 1999, the reports of the intermediate and final analyses of the trial Lyon Diet Heart Study; in 2003, a major epidemiological study in Greece showing a strong inverse association between a Mediterranean score and the risk of cardiovascular complications; in 2011-2012, several reports showing that even non-Mediterranean populations can gain benefits from long-term adhesion to the Mediterranean diet; and in 2013, the PREDIMED trial showing a significant risk reduction in a low-risk population. Contrary to the pharmacological approach of cardiovascular prevention, the adoption of the Mediterranean diet has been associated with a significant reduction in new cancers and overall mortality. Thus, in terms of evidence-based medicine, the full adoption of a modern version of the Mediterranean diet pattern can be considered one of the most effective approaches for the prevention of fatal and nonfatal CVD complications.

PMID: 24105822 [PubMed - indexed for MEDLINE]

And yes, all of your cardiovascular markers improve regardless of what macronutrients you eat, as long as weight is coming off. It's the weight loss alone that confers protection. Take a look at the studies below. It doesn't matter if you eat mostly fat, mostly carbs, no carbs, some protein, no protein… as long as you are in a calorie deficit, and you are losing weight, you will improve all of your cardiovascular markers!

Changes in weight loss, body composition and cardiovascular disease risk after altering macronutrient distributions during a regular exercise program in obese women

Chad M Kerksick, Jennifer Wismann-Bunn, Donovan Fogt, Ashli R Thomas, Lem Taylor, Bill I Campbell, Colin D Wilborn, Travis Harvey, Mike D Roberts, Paul La Bounty, Melyn Galbreath, Brandon Marcello, Christopher J Rasmussen & Richard B Kreider

Background

This study's purpose investigated the impact of different macronutrient distributions and varying caloric intakes along with regular exercise for metabolic and physiological changes related to weight loss.

Methods

One hundred forty-one sedentary, obese women (38.7 ± 8.0 yrs, 163.3 ± 6.9 cm, 93.2 ± 16.5 kg, 35.0 ± 6.2 kg·m⁻², 44.8 ± 4.2% fat) were randomized to either no diet + no exercise control group (CON) a no diet + exercise control (ND), or one of four diet + exercise groups (high-energy diet [HED], very low carbohydrate, high protein diet [VLCHP], low carbohydrate, moderate protein diet [LCMP] and high carbohydrate, low protein [HCLP]) in addition to beginning a 3x-week supervised resistance training program. After 0, 1, 10 and 14 weeks, all participants completed testing sessions which included anthropometric, body composition, energy expenditure, fasting blood samples, aerobic and muscular fitness assessments. Data were analyzed using repeated measures ANOVA with an alpha of 0.05 with LSD post-hoc analysis when appropriate.

Results

All dieting groups exhibited adequate compliance to their prescribed diet regimen as energy and macronutrient amounts and distributions were close to prescribed amounts. Those groups that followed a diet and exercise program reported significantly greater anthropometric (waist circumference and body mass) and body composition via DXA (fat mass and % fat) changes. Caloric restriction initially reduced energy expenditure, but successfully returned to baseline values after 10 weeks of dieting and exercising. Significant fitness improvements (aerobic capacity and maximal strength) occurred in all exercising groups. No significant changes occurred in lipid panel constituents, but serum insulin and HOMA-IR values decreased in the VLCHP group. Significant reductions in serum leptin occurred in all caloric restriction + exercise groups after 14 weeks, which were unchanged in other non-diet/non-exercise groups.

Conclusions

Overall and over the entire test period, all diet groups which restricted their caloric intake and exercised experienced similar responses to each other. Regular exercise and modest caloric restriction successfully promoted anthropometric and body composition improvements along with various markers of muscular fitness. Significant increases in relative energy expenditure and reductions in circulating leptin were found in response to all exercise and diet groups. Macronutrient distribution may impact circulating levels of insulin and overall ability to improve strength levels in obese women who follow regular exercise.

Regardless of what macronutrient breakdown you use, if you are losing weight, all of your cardiovascular risk factors improve

Take a look at another study (below) that was published in the New England Journal of Medicine. Regardless of which macronutrient you emphasize, your cardiovascular markers will all improve, so long as the diet you are following is actually causing weight loss.

N Engl J Med. Author manuscript; available in PMC 2009 Oct 19

https://www.ncbi.nlm.nih.gov/pmc/ar
ticles/PMC2763382/

Ctrl+Click to follow link

PMID: 19246357

Comparison of Weight-Loss Diets with Different Compositions of Fat, Protein, and Carbohydrates

Frank M. Sacks, M.D.,[1,2] George A. Bray, M.D.,[3] Vincent J. Carey, Ph.D.,[2] Steven R. Smith, M.D.,[3] Donna H. Ryan, M.D.,[3] Stephen D. Anton, Ph.D.,[3] Katherine McManus, M.S., R.D.,[1] Catherine M. Champagne, Ph.D.,[3] Louise M. Bishop, M.S., R.D.,[1] Nancy Laranjo, B.A.,[2] Meryl S. Leboff, M.D.,[1] Jennifer C. Rood, Ph.D.,[3] Lilian de Jonge, Ph.D.,[3] Frank L. Greenway, M.D.,[3] Catherine M. Loria, Ph.D.,[3] Eva Obarzanek, Ph.D.,[3] and Donald A. Williamson, Ph.D.[3]
Author information Copyright and License information Disclaimer
The publisher's final edited version of this article is available at N Engl J Med
See other articles in PMC that cite the published article

Associated Data
Supplementary Materials

Abstract

BACKGROUND

The possible advantage for weight loss of a diet that emphasizes protein, fat, or carbohydrates has not been established, and there are few studies that extend beyond 1 year.

METHODS

We randomly assigned 811 overweight adults to one of four diets; the targeted percentages of energy derived from fat, protein, and carbohydrates in the four diets were 20, 15, and 65%; 20, 25, and 55%; 40, 15, and 45%; and 40, 25, and 35%. The diets consisted of similar foods and met guidelines for cardiovascular health. The participants were offered group and individual instructional sessions for 2 years. The primary outcome was the change in body weight after 2 years in two-by-two factorial comparisons of low fat versus high fat and average protein versus high protein and in the comparison of highest and lowest carbohydrate content.

RESULTS

At 6 months, participants assigned to each diet had lost an average of 6 kg, which represented 7% of their initial weight; they began to regain weight after 12 months. By 2 years, weight loss remained similar in those who were assigned to a diet with 15% protein and those assigned to a diet with 25% protein (3.0 and 3.6 kg, respectively); in those assigned to a diet with 20% fat and those assigned to a diet with 40% fat (3.3 kg for both groups); and in those assigned to a diet with 65% carbohydrates and those assigned to a diet with 35% carbohydrates (2.9 and 3.4 kg, respectively) (P>0.20 for all comparisons). Among the 80% of participants who completed the trial, the average weight loss was 4 kg; 14 to 15% of the participants had a reduction of at least 10% of their initial body weight. Satiety, hunger, satisfaction with the diet, and attendance at group sessions were similar for all diets; attendance was strongly associated with weight loss (0.2 kg per session attended). The diets improved lipid-related risk factors and fasting insulin levels.

CONCLUSIONS

Reduced-calorie diets result in clinically meaningful weight loss regardless of which macronutrients they emphasize.

Conclusions on cardiovascular risk:

- Obesity and elevated BMI increase all inflammatory and cardiovascular risk factors
- Calorie deficit and weight loss improve all cardiovascular risk factors
- Macronutrient breakdown makes no difference
- Leaner individuals have less cardiovascular and all-cause mortality risk

Chapter 9

Where Do I Start?

Print off those two pages above and calculate your caloric needs and intake (or write on them). Put your information into MyFitnessPal like we described above and start tracking! You can download the PDF version of these pages and other resources on http://DrAlo.net/free .

In the first two weeks, you will realize quickly that you were eating way more calories than you thought you were eating. Most of my patients think they are eating only 1200-1400 calories per day, but when I go through their meals with them, they are eating in excess of 4000 calories per day, and in many cases over 5000.

Let's say you weigh 200 pounds and you start by eating 2000 calories per day (200 x 10) and eating 140g protein per day (200 x 0.7). You track and follow this plan for 3-4 weeks. Weight is coming off slowly, about 0.5-1.0% of your body weight, each week. That's perfect! You leave everything the same. If weight is coming off too quickly, increase your calories by 100-150 per day (in the form of carbs mainly) and try again. You don't want to lose weight too quickly either, because you will be losing muscle and not fat. You don't need to increase protein or fat, all adjustments are made by lowering or increasing carbs. We set protein and fat first, and just adjust carbs.

If after you start this out, you aren't losing any weight, you need to reduce calories by 100-150 per day. If you are losing 0.5-1.0% of your total body weight each week, then keep going.

Obviously, if you are on your period or close to it, your numbers may be off, but just stick with it and be patient. You'll be back on track by next week.

You have to do this for the next year or two. You don't want to lose weight overnight. You didn't gain weight overnight, and you shouldn't expect to lose it overnight. If you only have 20-30 pounds to lose, plan for 20-30 weeks. If you need to lose 50 or more, give yourself a year or more. Don't try to rush it. The slower you lose wight, the less muscle you will lose and the more fat you will lose. You will like how you look.

This is really the crux of it. If you don't want to track calories, go back and read the section on how to lose weight without tracking calories and watch the video on YouTube that goes with it.

You have to eat foods you enjoy and like. I can't stress this enough. If you eat food that you have been eating forever, you will be able to adhere to it better. The most important part of weight loss is adherence. If you try to do a super restrictive diet where you eat tons of things you hate or avoid foods you love, you will not be able to stick to it long enough. I see this every day. My patients start a diet where they cut out pop and pasta (the two Ps) and lose weight for a few weeks, but then can't maintain for very long and end up gaining it all back because they didn't learn how to lose weight while eating the foods that they enjoy.

What if you only enjoy double cheeseburgers and fries? Can you still lose weight? Sure, it is trickier and you will have to reduce your portion sizes. For example, a double cheeseburger from Five Guys is 840 calories. And an order of small fries is 530 calories. So, you are looking at 1370 total calories. That doesn't leave you very many calories to eat the rest of the day. But you will learn to budget your calories accordingly. For a shorter female that's only 140 pounds trying to get down to 128, the 1370 may already put her over her calorie limit.

You can cut the cheeseburger in half and not eat all the fries. That will reduce your caloric load and you still get to enjoy it.

Is it bad for your health to eat cheeseburgers and fries? As we discussed earlier, if weight is coming off, you will actually improve your health markers. Just make sure you are in a calorie deficit. If you are overweight or gaining weight, and have multiple risk factors, then this isn't a good option at all and can be dangerous. Make sure you are in a calorie deficit and are losing weight.

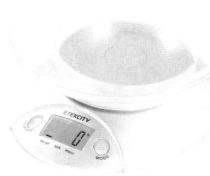

What If Your Tracking is Inaccurate?

I get this question a lot. A patient will tell me they tracked the chicken breast as 6 oz. but they aren't really sure. They didn't buy a food scale, and are guessing everything. Don't worry, it will still work! Why? Because we adjust your calories after a few weeks.

Let's say you are tracking inaccurately and are logging 2200 calories per day. Your weight hasn't changed in 4 weeks. We subtract 150 calories and now you are tracking 2050 calories and weight starts to come off. So, we will stick with this. It doesn't matter if the 2050 you are tracking is actually 1780 or 2350, it's working for you now, *in the way that you know how to track*. So, it's fine.

It's very helpful to use a food scale when you first start tracking, and track everything in grams. Your tracking will be way more accurate. Food scales can be purchased on Amazon for pretty cheap.

This is an example of a simple food scale. Learn to use these and track in grams. MyFitnessPal lets you change from ounces, to grams, to pounds, or whatever else you want to use.

Are there Medications That Help With Weight Loss?

Yes, there are a few approved, prescription obesity medications. You can discuss these with your physician and come up with a plan. I use these occasionally in my practice, but I have found that they aren't as helpful as we had previously hoped, mainly because people use them as a crutch. They should be used as a tool, and I spend a lot of time teaching my patients how to use them properly if we decide to use them. I also make sure they start tracking calories for a month before they even think about starting any meds. We usually use the medications as a last resort or as a booster in some scenarios. There have been some new meds approved that are quite promising for long term results. But we are getting beyond the scope of this book. For now, it's important to be aware of these options. You don't need them to get started.

Medication Interference

What about medications you are taking for other medical issues that can interfere with weight loss or weight gain? Take a look at the graphics below.

Weight loss Medications

- Metformin, symlin, acarbose, januvia/galvus, byetta, victoza, ACEIs/ARBs, Norvasc, topamax, wellbutrin, chemo, flagyl, amio, hydralazine, theophylline, fluoxetine, adderall, abilify, geodon, sulphasalazine, caffiene, acetazolamide, quinidine, amphotericine B,

Weight Gain Medications

- Diabetes: insulin, thiazolidinediones, and sulfonylureas
- Antipsychotics: haloperidol, clozapine, risperidone, quetiapine, olanzapine, and lithium
- Antidepressant: amitriptyline, imipramine, paroxetine, trazadone, alprazolam, and sertraline
- Epilepsy: valproate, carbamazepine, and gabapentin
- Steroids: prednisone or birth control pills
- Blood pressure: beta-blockers
- Antihistamines: ranitidine, diphenhydramine, cetirizine
- Opioids: oxycodone, hydrocodone

As you can see there are lots of commonly prescribed medications for other medical conditions that can also cause weight gain and or weight loss. If you are on something like this, you may want to talk to your physician about choosing different medications to help support your goals and medical conditions.

What are the most important factors when it comes to losing fat?

Keys To Fat Loss

- Keep calories as high as possible while still in a deficit

- Slow, maintained weight loss to protect lean mass (the slower the better)

- Don't lower fat too much (decreases testosterone and other hormones)

- Don't crash diet

- Calorie deficit

- Keep protein high

- Strength train hard

- Refeeds (results may vary)

- Diet Breaks (longer than refeeds)

The most important thing when it comes to losing fat is to keep calories as high as possible, while slowly and consistently losing weight. Don't be like my doctor friend that wanted a 240 pound male to eat 1200 calories per day. You need to eat as many calories as possible, while still causing weight loss. You also need to keep protein high. This makes you feel more full, protein is very satiating, and stimulates fat burning as well as muscle retention. This also helps keep your BMR higher. You don't want to drop your calories to 1200 if you are still losing at 1800. Why induce metabolic adaptation sooner?

Keep protein high! I can't tell you how many females I have seen eating only 30-40g of protein a day. Men aren't any better, usually eating 50-60g per day. You need your body weight x 0.7-1.6 in protein, or an average of 1g per pound. So, find ways to increase protein.

Strength training with heavy weights will send a signal to your body to hang on to muscle, and even build muscle. Studies have also found that when you lift weights while in a calorie deficit, most of your weight loss will come from fat stores, and not lean body mass. We need to keep that up.

Take diet breaks and refeeds as we discussed earlier. This increases your BMR and doesn't let you adapt to lower calories. And it's more satisfying and not as psychologically taxing. It helps, from a scientific standpoint, and a human behavior standpoint.

Chapter 10

What is Metabolic Adaptation?

My friend Amy was working out every day, lifting weights, walking, biking on weekends, and being very disciplined with eating. She was eating 1100 to 1200 calories per day. She was 5 foot 4 inches and weighed 175 pounds. She knows I'm the "weight loss doctor" so she stopped to talk about weight loss progress, or lack thereof. Weight loss had stopped. No matter what she did, she wasn't losing weight. At all. I looked over her food logs and she was super strict and accurate. She's the kind of person that weighed each "green grape" in grams and logged it. So, what's her problem? Why isn't she losing weight?

Does this sound familiar? So many people have been in a similar situation. This is normally called metabolic adaptation.

Metabolic adaptation is when your body adjusts to your current caloric intake and activity level. It reduces BMR and NEAT so that your weight loss comes to a screeching halt. Humans are able to adapt to very low caloric intakes. We want to avoid this situation.

TDEE/RMR/BMR goes down, and can stay down for very long time, sometimes, even years. The contestants on The Biggest Loser had their BMR depressed even 6 years after the contest was over. Prisoners of war survived for years on less than 500 calories per day. Hunter gatherer tribes can spend all day hunting for food, and their BMR and TDEE isn't all that different from ours. We adapt!

The Biggest Loser contestants were eating 1200 calories per day and exercising like crazy for 8 hours a day. They measured their BMR 6 years after the contest, and it was 25% lower than predicted. And of course, most gained all of their weight back and more.

Metabolic adaptation is a genetically programmed self-defense mechanism to ward off starvation and enhance weight gain/storage. It also reduces the chance of future diet success and enhances future weight regain.

With that said, your body has a buffer of 200-300 calories that it can use to keep your weight stable. So, if your maintenance calories are 2000, you can eat about 300 calories less or more than 2000 and your body will adjust your NEAT (non exercise activity thermogenesis) to keep your weight stable. As an example, if you ate 2300 calories, it may make you fidget around or walk and take more steps that day. If you ate 1700, it will reduce your imperceptible activity level to match. You will need to increase or decrease your calories by a lot more to really make a dent and get your weight moving in either direction. This is why you can have a bad day of eating and still stay on track.

Watch my Metabolic Adaptation video on YouTube as your assignment.

Welcome Back!

What Happens When You Hit a Real Plateau?

There are a few things you can do if your weight loss stops for 3-4 weeks. You haven't actually hit a plateau unless your weight loss stops for at least 4 weeks and you are being strict and compliant.

The first scenario is to stop your weight loss phase and take a diet break. Increase your calories back to maintenance and ride it out for 2 months. How do you know your maintenance? You have to increase calories by about 400-500 for men and usually 300 to 400 for women. Another way to do it is to slowly add back 150 calories a day and wait two weeks until weight stabilizes after the initial increase. Huh?

When you first increase calories, your muscles will take up glycogen and water will follow. You will see an initial increase in weight. Usually somewhere around 4-8 pounds. So, if you weigh180 pounds and get stuck at 180 pounds for 4 weeks while eating 2000 calories per day (strictly tracking), then increase your calories to 2300 and wait a few days (sometimes up to 2 weeks). Your weight will initially go up a few pounds (4-8 pounds) and then stabilize. Let's say you go up to 185, then it starts creeping back down again, increase your calories again in a week until your weight stabilizes. If your weight keeps creeping up, past that initial bump, you need to drop calories a bit. If you got to 2500 calories and your weight is still going up, take off 250 calories and maintain your weight.

Once you have figured this out, stay at this calorie count for 2 months. Diet breaks and maintenance phases help increase your metabolism, cause a higher percentage of weight loss to be from fat, protect against muscle loss, and improve diet adherence long term. When you lose weight slowly, you also break adaptations and habits that you have developed. Your body has a chance to reset and you don't get diet fatigue.

Be mindful that most people who aren't losing weight or get stuck, it's because they stopped tracking strictly or aren't counting bites, licks, and tastes (BLT). Make sure you are tracking strictly, or go back to tracking if you stopped, and see if it starts coming off again.

The second scenario is that you have not been losing weight for very long and you don't need a diet break, but weight loss has stopped. Assuming you are tracking calories strictly and you haven't gotten lax, what do you do in this scenario?

You can:

- Reduce calories slightly (fat or carbs, not protein)
- Add in more exercise or activity

- Lower carbs and fat by 5-10-15% per day (keep protein the same)
- Increase activity 5-10-15% (may not make a difference at all) *

*Relative to your current activity level

This can help get you back on track. But make sure you are actually tracking in the same way that you have been. A lot of people will track for 2-3 weeks then stop tracking and slowly and imperceptibly start eating slightly more (BLTs). As long as you are tracking in the same way you have been, it will be fine. Like we discussed earlier, even if you aren't tracking 100% accurately, as long as you are tracking consistently, it will still work.

Long Term Adherence

Because over 95% of people gain their weight back in 3-5 years, it's important to examine why some people don't gain their weight back. We don't want to be part of the 95%. Most Americans, over 70%, have lost significant weight. We all have that friend that lost 30 pounds then regained it. Heck, just read the first part of this book and look at my story. I have lost and regained the same 20-30 pounds over and over again. It's quite common. But we want to break that mold and figure out how to keep the weight off.

Studies have shown that there are five things that help you stick to your weight loss plan consistently.

- Cognitive Restraint in some form
- Self-monitoring
- Regular Exercise (formed good habits)
- Structured Programs
- Ability to focus on long term goals

Studies:

https://pubmed.ncbi.nlm.nih.gov/18268511-dietary-adherence-and-weight-loss-success-among-overweight-women-results-from-the-a-to-z-weight-loss-study/

https://pubmed.ncbi.nlm.nih.gov/16854220-dietary-and-physical-activity-behaviors-among-adults-successful-at-weight-loss-maintenance/?from_single_result=pmc1555605

https://pubmed.ncbi.nlm.nih.gov/22516488-successful-weight-loss-among-obese-us-adults/?from_single_result=pmc3339766

https://pubmed.ncbi.nlm.nih.gov/19587114-regular-exercise-attenuates-the-metabolic-drive-to-regain-weight-after-long-term-weight-loss/?from_single_result=pmc2739786

https://pubmed.ncbi.nlm.nih.gov/21677272-biologys-response-to-dieting-the-impetus-for-weight-regain/?from_single_result=pmc3174765

Let's talk about each of these individually.

Cognitive Restraint in Some Form

Studies have shown that people who can exercise some form of cognitive restraint are better at keeping weight off long term. What kind of restraint? It can be anything, sticking to a calorie count, sticking to an eating schedule and not deviating, eating between certain hours, avoiding certain foods, going sober, cutting out pop, and other examples. When you can restrain yourself, you are more disciplined and better at following through long term.

Self-Monitoring

People who kept the weight off long term were better at self-monitoring and adjusting. They were better at monitoring their weight, their caloric intake, their fitness levels, and even in their daily lives. They formed better habits. Even just monitoring your finances better, your ad spend, your employees at work. All of this leads to behavioral patterns that are conducive to sustained weight loss and weight maintenance.

Regular Exercise

Exercise is not necessary for weight loss, but studies have shown that people who are able to do some kind of exercise or activity daily and make it a part of their lives, were more committed to eating right. The 10,000 steps a day does increase your NEAT and helps to a certain degree, but that's not why this works. This works because you have gotten into a mindset where you are consistent and conscious of your overall health and daily habits. You are more in tune with living healthy.

It's also motivation. If you lift weights once a week, or bike, or anything, part of you doesn't want to eat poorly and undo all that effort you are putting in. I have had patients and clients say to me, "I'm going to skip the (insert high calorie option) today, because I worked out so much. I don't want to reverse all that progress."

Structured Programs

People who are great at incorporating structure and good habits into their daily lives are better at keeping weight off long term. If you are the type of person that has a morning routine, or eats only certain things at lunch, or works out at 5am every day, and reads before bed, then you are more likely to be able to keep weight off. This is because you are already good at forming good behavior patterns. Notice how "human behavior" keeps coming up in everything? Everything in life revolves around human behavior, especially food and activity patterns. Create good lifelong patterns and habits.

Ability to Focus on Long Term Goals

When you are able to focus on long term goals, you are better at keeping weight off. I told you that weight loss is hard and you need to lose the weight slowly. Fast weight loss leads to fast regain. Some people may not see progress fast enough and lose interest. But if you are capable of focusing on the long-term outcome, even though it may take over a year, then you will do well.

This is also true for almost anything in life. Being able to set long term goals and consistently work towards them will make you happier and more successful.

Bonus Material #1

Special Populations

There are some common groups of people that think that they cannot lose weight. I am asked these questions nearly every day. Sometimes patients and clients feel that they are a special case, and that they cannot lose weight like everyone else. Let's dispel these myths one by one. If you don't feel like reading this section, or you feel that you are not in one of these groups, the short answer is yes, everyone can lose weight with this strategy. The vast majority of people are not a unique case and should be able to lose weight like everyone else.

Can You Lose Weight if You are Diabetic?

Yes, you can still lose weight if you are diabetic. In fact, a large portion of studies done on weight loss have been done on diabetics. Many of these studies were cited above.

There are two kinds of diabetics. Type 1 diabetics require insulin and cannot live without insulin. They can not make insulin. They need injections. As they lose weight, they may require slightly less insulin. So make sure you are being followed by your doctor carefully and inform them that you plan to lose wight so they can check in on you frequently. As type 1 diabetics become more overweight, they may develop insulin resistance, which makes them also like a type 2 diabetic.

Type 2 diabetics can make tons of insulin, but they are resistant to the effects of it and need help. They usually start out by taking medications in pill form that can help them become more sensitive to the insulin they already make, reducing their insulin resistance, not absorb as much nutrients and glucose, secrete more insulin, and a whole host of other new mechanisms. As they gain weight and become obese, they may require insulin and hence end up somewhat like a type 1 diabetic. It's also important to tell your doctor that you plan to lose weight, because they will need to monitor you closely.

Make no mistake, weight loss in and of itself, will lower your blood sugar and improve your insulin resistance. Exercise helps with this as well. The point I am trying to make is that it's not necessarily important to eliminate carbs to lose weight as a diabetic. So many times a patient will go to diabetic educator or talk to a friend, and they are told to lower carb intake. So they lower carb intake. They see me next month and they haven't lost a single pound. In fact, they gained weight and now need more insulin and more medications to help control their diabetes. This is a travesty. Lower total calories and causing weight loss is what will improve your diabetes. This has been proven time and time again in multiple studies.

Take a look at one such study.

https://pubmed.ncbi.nlm.nih.gov/29466592/

Effect of Low-Fat vs Low-Carbohydrate Diet on 12-Month Weight Loss in Overweight Adults and the Association With Genotype Pattern or Insulin Secretion: The DIETFITS Randomized Clinical Trial

Christopher D Gardner [1], John F Trepanowski [1], Liana C Del Gobbo [1], Michelle E Hauser [1], Joseph Rigdon [2], John P A Ioannidis [1] [3] [4] [5], Manisha Desai [2] [3] [4] [5], Abby C King [1] [3]

Affiliations + expand

PMID: 29466592   PMCID: PMC5839290   DOI: 10.1001/jama.2018.0245
Free PMC article

Erratum in

Units of Measure Error.
[No authors listed]
JAMA. 2018 Apr 3;319(13):1386. doi: 10.1001/jama.2018.2977.
PMID: 29614160   Free PMC article.   No abstract available.

Incorrect Funding/Support Section.
[No authors listed]
JAMA. 2018 Apr 24;319(16):1728. doi: 10.1001/jama.2018.4854.
PMID: 29710144   Free PMC article.   No abstract available.

Abstract

Importance: Dietary modification remains key to successful weight loss. Yet, no one dietary strategy is consistently superior to others for the general population. Previous research suggests genotype or insulin-glucose dynamics may modify the effects of diets.

Objective: To determine the effect of a healthy low-fat (HLF) diet vs a healthy low-carbohydrate (HLC) diet on weight change and if genotype pattern or insulin secretion are related to the dietary effects on weight loss.

Design, setting, and participants: The Diet Intervention Examining The Factors Interacting with Treatment Success (DIETFITS) randomized clinical trial included 609 adults aged 18 to 50 years without diabetes with a body mass index between 28 and 40. The trial enrollment was from January 29, 2013, through April 14, 2015; the date of final follow-up was May 16, 2016. Participants were randomized to the 12-month HLF or HLC diet. The study also tested whether 3 single-nucleotide polymorphism multilocus genotype responsiveness patterns or insulin secretion (INS-30; blood concentration of insulin 30 minutes after a glucose challenge) were associated with weight loss.

Interventions: Health educators delivered the behavior modification intervention to HLF (n = 305) and HLC (n = 304) participants via 22 diet-specific small group sessions administered over 12 months. The sessions focused on ways to achieve the lowest fat or carbohydrate intake that could be maintained long-term and emphasized diet quality.

Main outcomes and measures: Primary outcome was 12-month weight change and determination of whether there were significant interactions among diet type and genotype pattern, diet and insulin secretion, and diet and weight loss.

Results: Among 609 participants randomized (mean age, 40 [SD, 7] years; 57% women; mean body mass index, 33 [SD, 3]; 244 [40%] had a low-fat genotype; 180 [30%] had a low-carbohydrate genotype; mean baseline INS-30, 93 µIU/mL), 481 (79%) completed the trial. In the HLF vs HLC diets, respectively, the mean 12-month macronutrient distributions were 48% vs 30% for carbohydrates, 29% vs 45% for fat, and 21% vs 23% for protein. Weight change at 12 months was -5.3 kg for the HLF diet vs -6.0 kg for the HLC diet (mean between-group difference, 0.7 kg [95% CI, -0.2 to 1.6 kg]). There was no significant diet-genotype pattern interaction (P = .20) or diet-insulin secretion (INS-30) interaction (P = .47) with 12-month weight loss. There were 18 adverse events or serious adverse events that were evenly distributed across the 2 diet groups.

Conclusions and relevance: In this 12-month weight loss diet study, there was no significant difference in weight change between a healthy low-fat diet vs a healthy low-carbohydrate diet, and neither genotype pattern nor baseline insulin secretion was associated with the dietary effects on weight loss. In the context of these 2 common weight loss diet approaches, neither of the 2 hypothesized predisposing factors was helpful in identifying which diet was better for whom.

Trial registration: clinicaltrials.gov Identifier: NCT01826591.

Read the conclusion if you don't want to go through the entire article. They tested a low fat versus a low carb diet in diabetics for weight loss. You can read the details. Both groups lose the same amount of weight (5.3 vs 6.0 kg)

Can I lose Weight If I Am Pregnant?

Pregnancy and the post-partum period pose special challenges when it comes to weight management.

The American College of Obstetrics and Gynecology no longer recommend massive amounts of weight gain during pregnancy. They have tamed their recommendations and are much more in tune with other medical groups. Here are their recommendations.

For most women:

If you are extremely obese (BMI over 40), they recommend not gaining any weight at all, and in fact they recommend losing weight during pregnancy.

If you are obese (BMI 30-39.9), they recommend weight gain of up to 10 pounds.

If you are overweight (BMI 25-29.9), they recommend modest gains of up to 5-20 pounds.

If you're in the normal weight range (BMI 18.5 to 24.9), they recommend weight gain of up to 25-30 pounds.

I you are underweight (BMI below 18.5), they recommend gaining as much as 28-40 pounds.

Whether you are pregnant now, or plan to be pregnant, or you have already given birth, the answer is yes. You can lose weight while pregnant. So many studies have been done on this and the biggest finding is that if you did "diet only" you lose more weight than the groups that did "activity only" and the group that added activity to diet (combined group).

You can read a very nice review of GWG (gestational weight gain) at:
https://pubmed.ncbi.nlm.nih.gov/26447010/

But one of the conclusions is:

"More specifically, dietary interventions were the most effective in reducing weight gain, with a mean weight loss of -3.84kg compared with -0.72kg and -1.06kg for physical activity and the mixed (diet plus physical activity) approach, respectively."

What about after pregnancy?

How can I get back to my original weight? That's the question that most people ask and want a magical answer. It's usually followed by, "And I still want to breastfeed."

You can still lose weight, eat right, and breastfeed. In fact, breastfeeding uses up a lot of mom's excess stored calories (fat) to help make milk. You can still follow everything we have discussed after giving birth. Pay special attention to hydration. To produce milk, you have to be well hydrated. Your body needs the fluids to make milk. If you are dehydrated your milk production (fat burning) process will shut down. Drink more water and you will make more milk (burn more fat). Of course, not everyone will lose weight from breastfeeding alone, you still have to be in a calorie deficit. Don't use breastfeeding as an excuse to eat excessive amount of food because you are "eating for two". I've heard that one plenty.

If you followed exactly what is in this book you will be able to lose weight before, after, and during pregnancy. Make sure you talk to your doctor first to make sure it is ok to go on a calorie restricted diet and start an exercise program.

I highly encourage you to watch my YouTube playlist on Weight Loss Before, During, and After Pregnancy:

Go do that now, it's not very long.

Welcome back!

Can I Lose Weight If My Thyroid is Off?

Your thyroid is not the reason you are overweight. If you have a weight problem, you have a weight problem. You've had it for a long time. Don't blame your thyroid! Thyroid problems can easily be addressed and treated by an endocrinologist. I highly recommend you are under the supervision of an endocrinologist and not an

Instagram "hormone specialist". If you actually have a hormone or thyroid problem, your endocrinologist or family doctor can get you balanced and stabilized. Please do not go online and search for home remedies. They can kill you if you have a serious problem.

We need to stop blaming our genetics, our spouses, our thyroids, our jobs and other factors for our weight problems. We are overweight, because we eat way more calories than we burn, and we haven't been able to get this under control.

A lot of people think that their thyroid is the reason that they are overweight. People who are hypothyroid (underactive thyroid) think that being underactive means that you will not be able to lose weight. The fact of the matter is that when you are hypothyroid, your body also decreases your appetite, so you don't eat as much. So, you will maintain your current weight.

People think that when they are hyperthyroid (overactive thyroid), they will lose weight. That's not true either. Hyperactive thryroids also increase your appetite and you eat more. Hence, you stay at your normal weight. Remember our bodies are very smart! They try to maintain our current weight at all costs.

If inducing hyperthryoidism was a way to lose weight, we'd be putting everyone on thyroid medication. Unfortunately, they have tried that, and it does not work. Further, there are a lot of problems with being hyperthyroid that are fatal. You heart can beat excessively fast, go into irregular rhythms, and ultimately go into heart failure. People have died from this.

On a related note, please make sure you are getting some iodized salt. Your body needs iodine to survive. You can not make thyroid hormones without iodine. Recently there has been a fad toward Himalayan salt and other forms of salt. It's fine, but please make sure you are getting enough iodine. You need this to live and make thyroid hormone, which increases your metabolism.

So How Do I Get My Kids to Lose Weight

Unfortunately, this is a new epidemic as you saw in the charts in the beginning of this book. Childhood obesity rates are nearing 20%. Our children are becoming mere copies of ourselves. Obesity is starting sooner and sooner and we are detecting diabetes and other diseases at a younger age. Entire books have been written on this topic, but unfortunately most take a very non-scientific approach to weight loss in kids.

One of the most important things to keep in mind is to avoid developing a bad relationship with food in your kids. You can't tell them that food is either "good" or "bad". Food is food. Some foods contain more carbs, some more, fats, and some more proteins. A donut is a carb fried in fat. Ice cream is mostly carbs and fat. Chicken nuggets are proteins, coated in carbs, fried in fat. All of these have nutritional value and a caloric cost associated with them. We have to teach kids proper budgeting of food and calories. If you want some ice cream, maybe cut out something else. Or eat half and take the rest home. Teach them the same way I am teaching you!

Another big issue with children and weight loss, is that you don't want to tell children that they are "fat". You want them to know that they are not as healthy as they can be and should be making better choices. You can encourage them to be more active and maybe even start a friendly competition seeing who can get in more steps, you or them. Make it fun!

You don't want it to become an image thing. They already have enough peers at school calling them "fat boy" and "big girl". Walking this fine line is a daunting task.

Starts at home

It all starts with the adults. People inherit bad eating habits, not obesity. The adults in the household should always cook and or bring home good wholesome meals and set good examples. There is no reason to stop by McDonald's on the way home and pick up fast food for dinner every single day. Sure, you can, but teach them that they can only eat half of it. Remember, if weight is coming off, their cardiovascular risk factors will improve. So, don't be afraid of "fast food" or "junk". Remember the Twinkie Diet? And the Five Guys example?

If mom and dad are eating too much, so will the kids. Follow these guidelines and make healthy choices. This starts as young as when children are 2 years old. They know what they like and can start requesting foods.

Get it out of the house

If your kids can't stop overeating calorie dense food, then don't bring that food home. Don't want your kids to eat chips? Get them out of the house. Don't buy it. Don't make it. Don't even introduce it to them. Unfortunately, the food industry has created highly palatable, very high calorie foods. Foods like Doritos, Oreos, Twinkies, ribs, fries and others are super good tasting, and you can't eat just one. Of course, I would prefer if you taught them portion control and self-control, but if your child is morbidly obese and your circumstances are such that you can't control them at all times, it may be necessary to not have that food in the house.

Reward good choices

When kids choose apple slices over fries, reward them with positive reinforcement. This always works. Kids will compete to see who can make the healthiest choices.

Educate

Kids aren't dumb. We find this out more and more every day. Talk to your kids about why healthy foods are better than bad ones. Discuss heart disease, vegetables, fruits, and why they are power foods. Kids will make better choices when they are equipped with better information. Have a family sit-down session and discuss various family foods and why they may or may not be good choices. Your kids may end up helping you avoid poor food choices.

Set an example

Nothing is more deflating than watching the leader not follow the rules. Kids love their parents, and love doing what their parents do. Always set a good example. If you order fries, but have them order apple slices, you are destroying the new paradigm from the inside out. When they go out alone, they will order fries. Set a good example at all times. Don't create a double standard. Healthy is healthy at any age.

Take it to the schools

Go to your school boards and make a difference. There is no reason why pizza, burgers, and fries should be the only food choices. Make sure that healthy alternatives are available and that your kids will only eat those foods. Don't be a pacifist about this. It's your children's life at stake. Go to the meetings and make them change their menu completely. Kids are more likely to adhere to good eating habits when they are surrounded by it on all fronts.

Play outside

There is no reason to sit around and watch television or play video games. Avoid television like the plague. If you can go outside and play, go outside and play. Play tag, play catch, play basketball, hide and seek, play any outdoor game. Anything is better than sitting around inside doing nothing. This will also help the adults become more active as well. If the weather isn't nice, sign up for a local recreational facility, YMCA, gym membership or anything that will allow you and your kids to participate in activities that involve movement.

Weight Loss Over 60

If you remember the metabolism section, over 60 is about when metabolism starts to slow down. But you still can lose weight. It's not all that different than weight loss below 60.

Weight loss can still be achieved at any age, but now you have to do specific things to increase your metabolism. Adding some weight training and resistance training to your regimen will go a long way toward helping increase your metabolism.

Take a look at the later bonus material for a full exercise and fitness program. Big compound movements like squats will build muscle which will increase your metabolism.

Try to get into a "young" frame of mind. Don't always avoid activities or outings because "I'm too old for that." Make sure your physician has cleared the activity, then go do it. Horseback riding, golfing, basketball, fishing, biking, weightlifting, body building, volleyball, softball, and soccer are all activities that you can enjoy at any age. Get into a young mindset and get active. If you have bad knees, bad hips, and other ailments, see a rehab and physical therapist and have them show you somethings that you are able to do.

PCOS and Weight Loss

Women with Polycystic Ovarian Syndrome can have cysts on their ovaries. But they are also insulin resistant and can have higher levels of testosterone. Is it harder to lose weight if you have PCOS? A large meta-analysis was done on this topic and published in 2017. Researchers looked at all studies (meta analysis) that compared weight loss in women with and without PCOS. Here is the study and some conclusions.

Weight Management Interventions in Women with and without PCOS: A Systematic Review

Josefin Kataoka [1] [2], Eliza C Tassone [3], Marie Misso [4], Anju E Joham [5], Elisabet Stener-Victorin [6], Helena Teede [7] [8], Lisa J Moran [9] [10]

Affiliations + expand
PMID: 28885578   PMCID: PMC5622756   DOI: 10.3390/nu9090996
Free PMC article

Abstract

Polycystic ovary syndrome (PCOS) is a common endocrinopathy among women associated with reproductive, metabolic and psychological features. While weight management is recommended as first-line treatment, it is unclear if women with PCOS achieve similar benefits as women without PCOS. This systematic review thus aimed to compare the efficacy of weight management interventions in women with and without PCOS. Databases were searched until May 2017. The primary outcome was weight and anthropometric, reproductive, metabolic and psychological measures were secondary outcomes. Of 3264 articles identified, 14 studies involving $n = 933$ ($n = 9$ high and $n = 5$ moderate risk of bias) met the inclusion criteria. No statistically significant differences in weight or weight loss following the intervention were found between women with and without PCOS in five studies, with the remaining studies not comparing the difference in weight or weight loss between these groups. Secondary outcomes did not differ significantly between the two groups. This review identified that there is a paucity of high quality research in this area and that more rigorous research is needed.

After finding studies that met the inclusion criteria, there was no difference in weight loss between women who had PCOS and women who did not have PCOS. Both groups were able to lose weight. When they looked at BMI changes between the two groups, they concluded, "Three studies reported a non-statistically significant difference in BMI between the two groups". This is a direct quote from the study.

I highly recommend looking at the charts and graphs in this article: https://www.ncbi.nlm.nih.gov/pmc/articles/PMC5622756/

Bonus Material #2

Exercise and Fitness

Once again, exercise is not necessary for weight loss, but it can help. There have been many studies showing no additional benefit to exercise in terms of weight loss alone. That energy balance alone (caloric intake) determines weight loss or weight gain. Yes, exercise is great for your health, and when done right, can help increase your metabolism, which will help tremendously. While you don't need exercise, I highly recommend it. Especially, if you are quite overweight. It will help improve appetite regulation. The more overweight you are, and the less active you are, the worse your appetite regulation.

We will discuss exercise prescriptions and I will give you a full exercise program that you can follow. You won't need anything else beyond what's in this book!

Exercise Modalities

There are four basic exercise modalities.

1. Endurance- Aerobic endurance training (Cardio)

2. Strength- Resistance training (Weights)

3. Balance

4. Flexibility

For our purposes, we will be discussing Endurance and Strength, not Balance and Flexibility. Balance and Flexibility are beyond the scope of this book. Sure, you can improve your balance and flexibility with many of the strength and endurance exercises that we discuss.

Cardio vs Weights

This is an age-old discussion. We need to understand how to properly use both for our health and fitness goals. They are different and cause different adaptations. You have to decide what your goals are so that you can select the proper exercise program to meet those goals.

If your goal is to just get into better shape and improve your overall health, then almost anything will work. Yes, anything! You can walk, run, swim, lift weights, bike, jog, hike, play basketball, golf, and do almost anything. Anything is better than nothing. If you are currently sedentary, find an activity you enjoy and start doing that. Your health and fitness will improve.

If you want to improve your cardiovascular mortality and all cause mortality, you can do more cardiovascular style workouts. Things like walking, jogging, running, hiking, swimming, and incline walking will all fit the bill. This will generally not help you grow your muscles or increase your BMR. Sure, your BMR will go up slightly because you started a new activity, but over time, your BMR can actually go down.

Your body can adapt to most forms of intense cardio. If you start jogging three miles a day, you may burn a lot of calories when you first start doing this, but as time goes on, your body adapts, and you improve your cardiorespiratory capacity, and you will burn fewer calories. Remember, we are not doing this for calorie burn or to create a deficit. This is just to fulfill your goal of improving your cardiovascular fitness level. And you will.

As a reference point, here is a chart showing how many calories you can burn doing various types of activities.

Calorie Expenditure 30 minutes Exercise

Activity Mode	110 lbs.	143 lbs.	187 lbs.	220 lbs.
Aerobic Dance	150	253	433	599
Moderate Cycling (12-13.9 mph)	184	311	531	735
Circuit Training	184	311	531	735
Bodybuilding/Powerlifting	139	232	397	551
Rowing: Moderate 100W	160	273	464	646
Running (10 min./mi.)	231	389	665	919
Running (7 min./mi.)	323	543	938	1286
Basketball Game	184	311	531	735
Boxing: Sparring	139	348	598	830
Soccer Game	231	389	665	919
Walking 3.0mph	76	130	219	305
Swimming Laps	231	389	665	919

Energy Expenditure (kcal/min) = (METs x 3.5 x Body Mass)/200

Hoffman, Jay. Norms for Fitness, Performance, and Health. Human Kinetics, 2006. [9] Hoffman, J. (2006). Norms for fitness, performance, and health. Champaign, IL: Human Kinetics.

If you weigh 110 pounds, you can burn 323 calories running for 30 minutes at a pace of 7 minute miles. If you weigh 220 pounds, you could burn 1286 calories doing that same thing. Walking at 3 mph burns the least amount of calories, and there is a whole lot in between. Biking, bodybuilding, and circuit training don't burn that many calories.

Remember, we are not doing these activities for the calorie burn. We are doing these because we enjoy them. It's just to get active. The best activity is the one you can do consistently long term. For most people, that will be walking.

Dangers of Excessive Cardio

Can you do too much cardio? Sure, excessive cardio has been shown to cause your heart muscles to remodel and your coronary arteries to harden faster than expected. You can read more about this in the

Mayo Clinic Proceedings article.
https://www.mayoclinicproceedings.org/article/S0025-6196(12)00473-9/fulltext

Here is a quick summary of the article:

Article Highlights

- People who exercise regularly have markedly lower rates of disability and a mean life expectancy that is 7 years longer than that of their physically inactive contemporaries. However, a safe upper-dose limit potentially exists, beyond which the adverse effects of exercise may outweigh its benefits.

- Chronic intense and sustained exercise can cause patchy myocardial fibrosis, particularly in the atria, interventricular septum, and right ventricle, creating a substrate for atrial and ventricular arrhythmias.

- Chronic excessive sustained exercise may also be associated with coronary artery calcification, diastolic dysfunction, and large-artery wall stiffening.

- Veteran endurance athletes in sports such as marathon or ultramarathon running or professional cycling have been noted to have a 5-fold increase in the prevalence of atrial fibrillation.

- Intense endurance exercise efforts often cause elevation in biomarkers of myocardial injury (troponin and B-type natriuretic peptide), which were correlated with transient reductions in right ventricular ejection fraction.

In another study, extreme marathoners had more calcium in their coronary arteries. Coronary Artery Calcium (CAC) score is an indicator of future heart attacks and strokes.

> Eur Heart J. 2008 Aug;29(15):1903-10. doi: 10.1093/eurheartj/ehn163. Epub 2008 Apr 21.

Running: the risk of coronary events : Prevalence and prognostic relevance of coronary atherosclerosis in marathon runners

Stefan Möhlenkamp [1], Nils Lehmann, Frank Breuckmann, Martina Bröcker-Preuss, Kai Nassenstein, Martin Halle, Thomas Budde, Klaus Mann, Jörg Barkhausen, Gerd Heusch, Karl-Heinz Jöckel, Raimund Erbel, Marathon Study Investigators; Heinz Nixdorf Recall Study Investigators

Affiliations + expand

PMID: 18426850   DOI: 10.1093/eurheartj/ehn163

Abstract

Aims: To quantify the prevalence of coronary artery calcification (CAC) in relation to cardiovascular risk factors in marathon runners, and to study its role for myocardial damage and coronary events.

Methods and results: In 108 apparently healthy male marathon runners aged >or=50 years, with >or=5 marathon competitions during the previous three years, the running history, Framingham risk score (FRS), CAC, and presence of myocardial late gadolinium enhancement (LGE) were measured. Control groups were matched by age (8:1) and FRS (2:1) from the Heinz Nixdorf Recall Study. The FRS in marathon runners was lower than in age-matched controls (7 vs. 11%, P < 0.0001). However, the CAC distribution was similar in marathon runners and age-matched controls (median CAC: 36 vs. 38, P = 0.36) and higher in marathon runners than in FRS-matched controls (median CAC: 36 vs. 12, P = 0.02). CAC percentile values and number of marathons independently predicted the presence of LGE (prevalence = 12%) (P = 0.02 for both). During follow-up after 21.3 +/- 2.8 months, four runners with CAC >or= 100 experienced coronary events. Event-free survival was inversely related to CAC burden (P = 0.018).

Conclusion: Conventional cardiovascular risk stratification underestimates the CAC burden in presumably healthy marathon runners. As CAC burden and frequent marathon running seem to correlate with subclinical myocardial damage, an increased awareness of a potentially higher than anticipated coronary risk is warranted.

I am not trying to scare you. The point of this is that anything taken to an extreme can be dangerous. If you want to run recreationally, don't go extreme. You will reap all the benefits of cardiovascular activity.

One drawback to doing a "cardio only" program, is that you will lose weight. Yes, you will lose weight. Not just fat. You will lose lean body mass too. You will lose muscle. If that's ok with you, it's fine. Proceed.

But please don't eat back calories that your fitness tracker tells you that you burned. Create a calorie deficit with food only. Your body will reduce NEAT and BMR and you will not burn as many calories as you think you are burning.

Remember this graph?

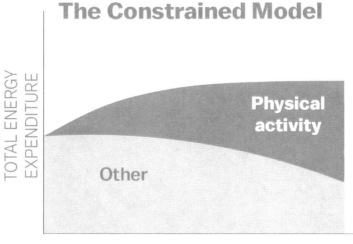

The Constrained Model

TOTAL ENERGY EXPENDITURE

Physical activity

Other

PHYSICAL ACTIVITY

SOURCE: Current Biology (2016)

There's an upper limit to how much calories you can burn with activity. So, keep that in mind. It's not limitless. You can only burn so many calories with physical labor. You can't run off thousands of calories a day.

If your goals are to get lean, build muscle, and get toned, then you will want to incorporate weightlifting or resistance training into your fitness program. Weightlifting increases BMR over time, because you build muscle. You will get stronger, and strength translates into everything! You will increase muscle cross sectional area, get stronger, and be able to do more. All of these adaptations, lead to increases in BMR.

When your BMR goes up, you will need to eat more food to sustain it. Or if you are trying to lose weight, and eat the same number of calories, you will actually lose weight. Let's say your BMR or TDEE is 2000 calories and your weight has been stable. An increase in your BMR (with weightlifting), will cause your weight to go down. Even though you are still eating 2000 calories per day. You'll lose weight even when you sleep.

Studies vary significantly in how much each additional pound of muscle raises your BMR. On the low end, each additional pound of muscle increases your BMR by 6-8 calories. On the higher end, studies demonstrated an increase of 50-80 calories. In reality, the number doesn't matter that much. Your body will need more calories, and you will look better in the end.

This goes for men and women. Women, you will not get bulky and look like a man. This is a huge myth. You are going to lose weight and get 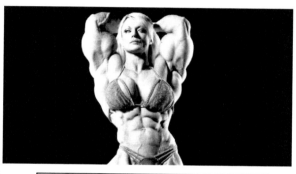 lean and toned. Those huge body builder women usually take

You aren't going to look like this!

steroids or have done some very extreme things to look like that. We are not asking you to do that. You will never look like that.

And that's the best thing about weightlifting. Your BMR will increase, and you can eat more and do less to lose weight. It's like magic.

Take a look at this study and the graphs that go with it.

Aerobic or Resistance Exercise, or Both, in Dieting Obese Older Adults

Dennis T Villareal[1], Lina Aguirre[1], A Burke Gurney[1], Debra L Waters[1], David R Sinacore[1], Elizabeth Colombo[1], Reina Armamento-Villareal[1], Clifford Qualls[1]

Affiliations

•PMID: 28514618
•PMCID: PMC5602187
•DOI: 10.1056/NEJMoa1616338
Free PMC article

Abstract

Background: Obesity causes frailty in older adults; however, weight loss might accelerate age-related loss of muscle and bone mass and resultant sarcopenia and osteopenia.

Methods: In this clinical trial involving 160 obese older adults, we evaluated the effectiveness of several exercise modes in reversing frailty and preventing reduction in muscle and bone mass induced by weight loss. Participants were randomly assigned to a weight-management program plus one of three exercise programs - aerobic training, resistance training, or combined aerobic and resistance training - or to a control group (no weight-management or exercise program). The primary outcome was the change in Physical Performance Test score from baseline to 6 months (scores range from 0 to 36 points; higher scores indicate better performance). Secondary outcomes included changes in other frailty measures, body composition, bone mineral density, and physical functions.

Results: A total of 141 participants completed the study. The Physical Performance Test score increased more in the combination group than in the aerobic and resistance groups (27.9 to 33.4 points [21% increase] vs. 29.3 to 33.2 points [14% increase] and 28.8 to 32.7 points [14% increase], respectively; P=0.01 and P=0.02 after Bonferroni correction); the scores increased more in all exercise groups than in the control group (P<0.001 for between-group comparisons). Peak oxygen consumption (milliliters per kilogram of body weight per minute) increased more in the combination and aerobic groups (17.2 to 20.3 [17% increase] and 17.6 to 20.9 [18% increase], respectively) than in the resistance group (17.0 to 18.3 [8% increase]) (P<0.001 for both comparisons). Strength increased more in the combination and resistance groups (272 to 320 kg [18% increase] and 288 to 337 kg [19% increase], respectively) than in the aerobic group (265 to 270 kg [4% increase]) (P<0.001 for both comparisons). Body weight decreased by 9% in all exercise groups but did not change significantly in the control group. Lean mass decreased less in the combination and resistance groups than in the aerobic group (56.5 to 54.8 kg [3% decrease] and 58.1 to 57.1 kg [2% decrease], respectively, vs. 55.0 to 52.3 kg [5% decrease]), as did bone mineral density at the total hip (grams per square centimeter; 1.010 to 0.996 [1% decrease] and 1.047 to 1.041 [0.5% decrease], respectively, vs. 1.018 to 0.991 [3% decrease]) (P<0.05 for all comparisons). Exercise-related adverse events included musculoskeletal injuries.

Conclusions: Of the methods tested, weight loss plus combined aerobic and resistance exercise was the most effective in improving functional status of obese older adults. (Funded by the National Institutes of Health; LITOE ClinicalTrials.gov number, NCT01065636.).

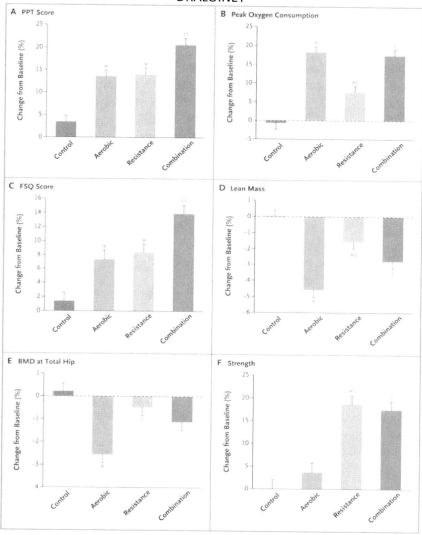

Look at the middle right graph. It shows lean body mass decreased with Aerobic (cardio) training. That means they lost muscle. We don't want to lose muscle. Unfortunately, cardio can cause a significant amount of lean body mass reduction. Sure, lean body mass decreased slightly with resistance training as well, but these were not weightlifters eating in a calorie surplus and eating enough protein. When you are in a calorie deficit, you will lose both fat and lean body mass. That's why we stress resistance training and eating sufficient protein, to try and mitigate muscle loss.

Look at the graph on the bottom left. This is Bone Mineral Density at the Hip. Aerobic training caused a significant amount of BMD loss at the hip. This is the last thing we need. I have seen too many little old ladies with broken hips. This can happen to men as well, but women usually are deficient in bone mineral density because of years of menstruation.

Finally, look at the bottom right graph. Strength increased the most with resistance training and this is very important. Strength translates into everything. Some of my patients don't have the strength to get up out of chair, this is very crucial for them.

Strength improves quality of life. Imagine being able to carry the water bottles from Costco into your car by yourself? Or put away that bowl above your head in the cupboard. Or lift that car engine up without help? Or carry all your books? Build a shed?

We will get into details of the exercise program later on. But just keep all of these things in mind.

The next study shows that slower rates of weight loss in elite athletes caused less muscle loss.

Effect of two different weight-loss rates on body composition and strength and power-related performance in elite athletes

Ina Garthe, Truls Raastad, Per Egil Refsnes, Ana Koivisto, Jorunn Sundgot-Borgen
Affiliations
•PMID: 21558571
•DOI: 10.1123/ijsnem.21.2.97

Abstract
When weight loss (WL) is necessary, athletes are advised to accomplish it gradually, at a rate of 0.5-1 kg/wk. However, it is possible that losing 0.5 kg/wk is better than 1 kg/wk in terms of preserving lean body mass (LBM) and performance. The aim of this study was to compare changes in body composition, strength, and power during a weekly body-weight (BW) loss of 0.7% slow reduction (SR) vs. 1.4% fast reduction (FR). We hypothesized that the faster WL regimen would result in more detrimental effects on both LBM and strength-related performance. Twenty-four athletes were randomized to SR (n = 13, 24 ± 3 yr, 71.9 ± 12.7 kg) or FR (n = 11, 22 ± 5 yr, 74.8 ± 11.7 kg). They followed energy-restricted diets promoting the predetermined weekly WL. All athletes included 4 resistance-training sessions/wk in their usual training regimen. The mean times spent in intervention for SR and FR were 8.5 ± 2.2 and 5.3 ± 0.9 wk, respectively (p < .001). BW, body composition (DEXA), 1-repetition-maximum (1RM) tests, 40-m sprint, and countermovement jump were measured before and after intervention. Energy intake was reduced by 19% ± 2% and 30% ± 4% in SR and FR, respectively (p = .003). BW and fat mass decreased in both SR and FR by 5.6% ± 0.8% and 5.5% ± 0.7% (0.7% ± 0.8% vs. 1.0% ± 0.4%/wk) and 31% ± 3% and 21 ± 4%, respectively. LBM increased in SR by 2.1% ± 0.4% (p < .001), whereas it was unchanged in FR (-0.2% ± 0.7%), with significant differences between groups (p < .01). In conclusion, data from this study suggest that athletes who want to gain LBM and increase 1RM strength during a WL period combined with strength training should aim for a weekly BW loss of 0.7%.

Which is why we want to lose weight in a slow and sustained manner. Not fast.

To summarize what we know about resistance training:

- Resistance training is much more effective than cardio (increases BMR)

- Explosive runs/sprints are comparable to resistance training

- Especially true for women and people with low metabolism

Advantages of weight training over cardio

- Anyone can weight lift, not everyone can run or swim

- Increases BMR

- Improves strength

- Improves mobility

- Improves quality of life

- Improves body composition

- Improves functionality

Many of you may have seen these graphics online. They illustrate the differences in body composition between people who focus on restricting calories severely and only do cardio versus a different cohort that eats sufficiently and lifts weights.

THE KEY TO LOSING FAT IS
LIFTING WEIGHTS!

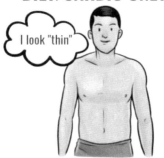 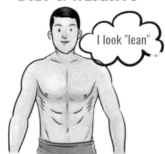

Obviously, this applies to men and women.

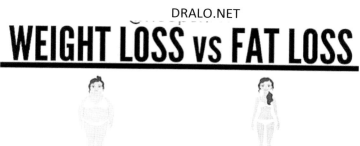

150 pounds
35% body fat

150 pounds
20% body fat

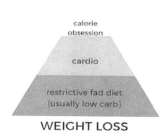

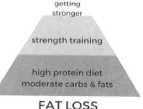

WEIGHT LOSS

FAT LOSS

What's My Exercise Prescription?

For the vast majority of my patients, I have them start somewhere. Anywhere. Something simple and doable. My patients aren't usually very healthy and many aren't capable of adopting a complex exercise regimen. Let's address them first before we move on to younger and healthier patients and clients.

The first step is to get clearance from your doctor to start an exercise regimen and calorie restricted diet. Make sure all of your medical conditions are taken care of and you are able to perform physical activity safely.

The most important thing if you are 200+ pounds overweight and have multiple medical issues is to start with calorie restriction. You have to get your calories down to something close to body weight X

10. If you are 360 pounds, you need to be at or around 3600 calories. It's nearly impossible to be active when you weigh so much. Start by walking. Just get up and walk around your house and even down the street. Take breaks if you have to. If you can't do more than one minute at a time, that's ok. Start by walking one minute and then resting. Do this at least 5 to 10 times per day. Then you can progress from there.

If you are 200 pounds overweight, but are quite fit and can exercise and lifts weights, you can skip to the Exercise and Fitness Program.

If you are 100-199 pounds overweight, you can start by walking 10-15 minutes per day. Break it up if you have to like above, but try to do this at least 3 times per day. Of course, you need to be eating body weight X 10 in calories. That goes without say. And make sure your medical conditions are well controlled. As you lose weight and are in better shape, you can skip ahead to the Exercise and Fitness program.

If you are 99 pounds or less overweight, you can start by restricting calories as above and jump right into the program below, if you are capable and cleared by your doctor.

Bonus Material #3

The Exercise & Fitness Program

Once again, you do not have to do this to achieve your weight loss goals, but you will like the way you look more if you do this. Exercise also helps increase your metabolism (if I haven't said this enough).

The program is designed to be an easy, one day per week, full-body program. As you become more advanced and stop seeing progress, or if your schedule allows, you can increase it to two or three days per week. But there is no reason to increase it if you are still seeing progress. We want the minimum effective dose (just like medicine). Why work out 2 days per week, if you are still seeing results with 1 day?

The program is composed of mainly compound lifts. Compound lifts are large movements that use more than one joint to perform the lift. Each lift is nearly a full body workout if done correctly. When you squat, you also train your core, your lats, your arms, and other muscle groups, not just your legs. When you bench press you are engaging your core, your legs, your triceps, deltoids, and multiple other body parts. They are large, multi-joint movements.

The Beginner and Intermediate level programs are the same, except that you do it more often per week in the Intermediate level.

The Beginner Program is once a week. As an Example, we use Monday. On Monday you would go to the gym, or your home gym and do the exercises listed below. You do two sets of each, unless otherwise listed.

Phase 1 is an 8 week program to get your muscles warmed up and ready to go. It's lighter weight than usual, just so you can get used to the movements and not get injured if your form isn't right. You select a weight that you can do 8 to 12 reps. This means that by the 10th or 11th rep, you are really struggling. It's ok if you manage to squeeze out 14 reps. But definitely don't make it so heavy that you are struggling to put up 3 reps. That comes later.

The 8 to 12 rep range is called "hypertrophy range". The weight you select is not so heavy that you can barely do 3 reps and not so light that you can do 20 or more reps. Hypertrophy means muscle growth. We start with this because it's lighter and safer and we want you to get your form down. In fact, if you want to lower the weight even more and select

Women

Do women do the same exercises as men? Yes, these are the best exercises for all genders. Anyone selling you a "women's program" is probably just fooling you. All genders benefit equally from compound lifts. The same lifts. There is nothing special or magical for different genders. If after you have lost tons of weight, you decide you want to emphasize more chest or more glutes, you can do more sets for those muscles and increase the frequency (number of days per week you do those exercises).

As an example, if you want to grow chest, you can bench press Monday, Wednesday, and Friday. If you want to grow glutes, you can do stiff legged deadlifts, or hip thrusts Monday Wednesday, and Friday. You get the idea. Increase frequency. It's the same exercises. But that's probably beyond the scope of this book, maybe a later book or cheatsheet will be available on these topics. Always check https://dralo.net for updates.

a weight that you can do 15-20 reps for the first 2 weeks, that's ok too. Do that until you feel comfortable.

Start each workout with a warmup on a bike, or jump rope, or jumping jacks, or air squats. Just do it for 30 seconds or a minute to get your heart pumping and blood flowing. This will help prevent injury.

Do a warmup set with just the bar, or no weight to get blood flowing to the muscles that you plan on using. So, before you do bench press, press the bar with no weight on it or do some pushups. Before squatting, do body weight squats or just squat the bar. This will prevent injury and get blood flowing to the proper muscles and get the ligaments stretched out and ready.

Phase 2 is also 8 weeks, but now that you have the movements down, we want you to increase the weight and select a weight that you can only do 4-6 reps. This is called "strength range" reps. This will increase your strength. You do the same exact exercises on Monday, the same way you did before, but now the weight is heavier.

Phase 3 is going back to hypertrophy range weight. After the 2 months of strength, you go a little lighter, and do 8-12 reps. You will notice that the weight is now heavier. When you first started, you could only bench 125 pounds for 8-12 reps. But after finishing a strength phase, you can now do 145 pounds for 8-12 reps. That's the whole idea and that's what we call "progressive overload". Slowly increase your weights and make it slightly harder. This obviously has a limit and you can't keep going up forever, otherwise we would all be benching 5000 pounds. Just try to progressively overload over time.

Do you have to do a strength phase? If you don't want to increase the weight or feel unsafe, it's ok. You don't have to. Just stick with the 8-12 rep range and slowly increase the weight over time. You'll still be fine.

Phase 4 would be cycling back to a strength phase. You get the idea. Every 8 weeks or so, you switch back to the phase that you haven't done.

Below is a page borrowed from my Weight Loss 101 Masterclass (DrAlo.net/weightloss), feel free to print it out and use it. Click the link to learn more about the class.

Exercise Program DrAlo.net

Warm Up: Two minutes on bike or jumping jacks

Beginner

Phase 1: (8 weeks)

Every Monday:
Squat 2 sets, 8-12 reps
Stiff Leg Deadlift: 2 sets, 8-12 reps
Walking Lunges: 10 back and forth
Bench 2 sets, 8-12 reps
Incline Bench: 2 sets, 8-12 reps
Overhead Press: 2 sets, 8-12 reps
Deadlifts 2 sets, 8-12 reps
Barbell Row: 2 sets, 8-12 reps
Pull-ups: AMRAPS (as many reps as possible)
Seated Cable Row: 2 sets, 8-12 reps
Lat Pull Down: 2 sets, 8-12 reps

Phase 2: (8 weeks)

Every Monday:
Squat 2 sets, 4-6 reps
Stiff Leg Deadlift: 2 sets, 4-6 reps
Walking Lunges: 10 back and forth
Bench 2 sets, 4-6 reps
Incline Bench: 2 sets, 4-6 reps
Overhead Press: 2 sets, 4-6 reps
Deadlifts 2 sets, 4-6 reps
Barbell Row: 2 sets, 4-6 reps
Pull-ups: AMRAPS (as many reps as possible)
Seated Cable Row: 2 sets, 4-6 reps
Lat Pull Down: 2 sets, 4-6 reps

Phase 3: (8 weeks)

Go back and repeat Phase 1 again with weights in the 8-12 rep range. Keep cycling back and forth between 4-6 and 8-12.

Intermediate

Phase 1: (12 weeks)

Every Monday, Wednesday, Friday:
Squat 2 sets, 8-12 reps
Stiff Leg Deadlift: 2 sets, 8-12 reps
Walking Lunges: 10 back and forth
Bench 2 sets, 8-12 reps
Incline Bench: 2 sets, 8-12 reps
Overhead Press: 2 sets, 8-12 reps
Deadlifts 2 sets, 8-12 reps
Barbell Row: 2 sets, 8-12 reps
Pull-ups: AMRAPS (as many reps as possible)
Seated Cable Row: 2 sets, 8-12 reps
Lat Pull Down: 2 sets, 8-12 reps

Phase 2: (12 weeks)

Every Monday, Wednesday, Friday:
Squat 2 sets, 4-6 reps
Stiff Leg Deadlift: 2 sets, 4-6 reps
Walking Lunges: 10 back and forth
Bench 2 sets, 4-6 reps
Incline Bench: 2 sets, 4-6 reps
Overhead Press: 2 sets, 4-6 reps
Deadlifts 2 sets, 4-6 reps
Barbell Row: 2 sets, 4-6 reps
Pull-ups: AMRAPS (as many reps as possible)
Seated Cable Row: 2 sets, 4-6 reps
Lat Pull Down: 2 sets, 4-6 reps

Phase 3: (12 weeks)

Go back and repeat Phase 1 again with weights in the 8-12 rep range. Keep cycling back and forth between 4-6 and 8-12.

These are mostly compound movements and a great place to start. Compound movements are big, multi joint movements that are almost full body workouts and really tax your body.

WEIGHT LOSS 101

If you want to see exercise demonstrations, take a look at my YouTube video explaining my workout. I will warn you, my workout routine is not the Beginner or Intermediate level one. I follow a Push Pull Legs routine which is explained in the video. It's almost the same exercises, but way more frequently and I don't do full body each day. I do legs one day, back one day (pull), and chest another day (push). That's called a push pull legs split. You are welcome to watch the video explaining it and decide to follow that routine after you finish the Beginner and Intermediate program.

Watch my YouTube video explaining these workouts, the philosophy, and the exercise demonstrations. Go watch it now and come back.

https://www.youtube.com/watch?v=FD7yIOeSplQ

If you want the full resolution 8.5 X 11 PDF for **my personal routine**, you can grab it here for free: https://dralo.net/exercise

For my very sedentary and overweight patients, I usually have them:

- Include cardio and resistance training

- Start at appropriate intensity

- Start with more cardio in beginning

- Transition to more resistance over time

- Weights increase over time

- Adapt over time

One last time, in case you missed it. Diet is way more important that exercise. Take a look at this study again if you glossed over it the first time.

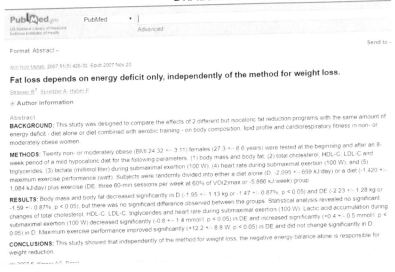

Ann Nutr Metab. 2007;51(5):428-32. Epub 2007 Nov 20.

Fat loss depends on energy deficit only, independently of the method for weight loss.

Strasser B[1], Spreitzer A, Haber P.
+ Author information

Abstract
BACKGROUND: This study was designed to compare the effects of 2 different but isocaloric fat reduction programs with the same amount of energy deficit - diet alone or diet combined with aerobic training - on body composition, lipid profile and cardiorespiratory fitness in non- or moderately obese women.

METHODS: Twenty non- or moderately obese (BMI 24.32 +/- 3.11) females (27.3 +/- 6.6 years) were tested at the beginning and after an 8-week period of a mild hypocaloric diet for the following parameters: (1) body mass and body fat, (2) total cholesterol, HDL-C, LDL-C and triglycerides, (3) lactate (millimol/liter) during submaximal exertion (100 W), (4) heart rate during submaximal exertion (100 W), and (5) maximum exercise performance (watt). Subjects were randomly divided into either a diet alone (D, -2,095 +/- 659 kJ/day) or a diet (-1,420 +/- 1,084 kJ/day) plus exercise (DE, three 60-min sessions per week at 60% of VO(2)max or -5,866 kJ/week) group.

RESULTS: Body mass and body fat decreased significantly in D (-1.95 +/- 1.13 kg or -1.47 +/- 0.87%, p < 0.05) and DE (-2.23 +/- 1.28 kg or -1.59 +/- 0.87%; p < 0.05), but there was no significant difference observed between the groups. Statistical analysis revealed no significant changes of total cholesterol, HDL-C, LDL-C, triglycerides and heart rate during submaximal exertion (100 W). Lactic acid accumulation during submaximal exertion (100 W) decreased significantly (-0.8 +/- 1.4 mmol/l, p < 0.05) in DE and increased significantly (+0.4 +/- 0.5 mmol/l, p < 0.05) in D. Maximum exercise performance improved significantly (+12.2 +/- 8.8 W, p < 0.05) in DE and did not change significantly in D.

CONCLUSIONS: This study showed that independently of the method for weight loss, the negative energy balance alone is responsible for weight reduction.

The study concludes that weight loss depended on calorie deficit alone. The group that did aerobic training plus diet did not lose any more weight than the group that did diet only. So please, please get your diet right first. There is no way to cause weight loss if you haven't controlled your diet. Please don't think that starting an exercise program will fix everything. It may for a little while, but then you will be back where you started.

Calories Out

This is the amount of energy you can "expend" or burn every day. It is not that easy to change this by very much. If you remember the chart we showed in the beginning, EAT (exercise activity thermogenesis) is only about 5% of TDEE. You can only increase or decrease this by so much, and it's capped, as we have shown previously.

Summary of Calories Out:

- Very difficult to change this

- Don't eat back calories that you burn off

- Calories and exercise should be independent factors

- We really don't know how much we are burning off and it is usually capped

Body Recomposition (gaining muscle while losing fat) is possible in four types of individuals.

These four groups of people can gain muscle and lose fat at the same time in a calorie deficit. And you probably fit into one of these categories.

- Obese

- New to training

- Deconditioned Lifters

- Anabolic steroids

The vast majority of us fit into the first three categories and should be able to see muscle gain and fat loss at the same time without having to go on dedicated bulking and cutting cycles. Advanced lifters and bodybuilders have to cycle between gaining muscle (bulking) and weight loss phases (cutting). As you get leaner, it will be harder to recomposition. That's beyond the scope of this book and can be explored later. Always check https://dralo.net for more information and more advanced techniques.

Weight Loss Summary

The below pyramid is from my Weight Loss 101 Masterclass and visually explains the foundations of weight loss. The most important layer is the foundation, this is your energy balance (calories). If you are consuming too many calories, nothing above that level can help you. The next most important step is eating enough protein to support fat loss and muscle retention (and even growth). The next level is to lift weights to also help retain muscle mass and even grow muscle while in a calorie deficit. The next level is to get your medical conditions right. This is a perquisite to weight loss and exercise and needs to be tuned up and adjusted as you lose weight. People who have hypertension and diabetes will need their medications adjusted as weight starts coming off.

The final phase of weight loss will be cardio. Physique athletes generally save cardio for the last few weeks before a bodybuilding show to burn off the final layers of fat, especially if they can't lower their calories any further or can't stop overeating.

For the vast majority of people, you can change this around and make these into pillars holding up a home. The home is fitness, and you need all of these components to hold up the home.

Fat Loss Pyramid

DrAlo.net

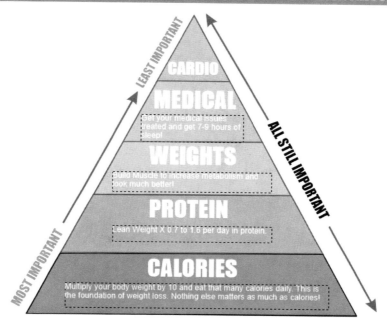

LEAST IMPORTANT

CARDIO

MEDICAL
Get your medical issues treated and get 7-9 hours of sleep!

WEIGHTS
Build Muscle to increase metabolism and look much better!

PROTEIN
Lean Weight X 0.7 to 1.6 per day in protein.

CALORIES
Multiply your body weight by 10 and eat that many calories daily. This is the foundation of weight loss. Nothing else matters as much as calories!

MOST IMPORTANT

ALL STILL IMPORTANT

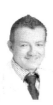

Everything is built on a foundation of a calorie deficit. You have to be in a calorie deficit to lose weight. You also need enough protein to support your weight loss goals, protect lean body mass, improve satiety, and stimulate fat loss. Lift weights to protect lean mass from being lost and to build more lean body mass. Get all of your serious medical issues taken care of (you could even put this first) and get enough sleep to recuperate and recover. Do cardio to protect your heart twice a week.

WEIGHT LOSS 101

Final Words

Conclusion

You now have everything you need to lose weight properly. This is **Actual Weight Loss**. There are no shortcuts or gimmicks. This is the best way to lose weight slowly, sustainably, safely, and permanently.

Weight loss isn't easy and there are so many things in life fighting against you. You have to tough it out and get through it. If you put your mind to it and make a few changes in your eating habits and start an exercise and fitness program, you should be set.

If you have more questions and need more information, check out the section below.

Resources

Now that you have finished this book, you should be well on your way to losing weight. If you need help, please don't hesitate to reach out. Shoot me an email or go to my website!

At my website you can download tons of free content, read articles, and sign up for classes!
https://DrAlo.net

Or shoot me an email:
MohammedAlo@gmail.com

Don't forget to watch my Weight Loss Playlist on YouTube:
https://www.youtube.com/watch?v=oLvjajxKnCw&list=PLj6vNKDa793E7_INCeuCanF1lVE-PK_nV

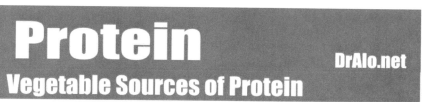

Protein
DrAlo.net

Vegetable Sources of Protein

Seitan
Tofu, Tempeh, Edamame
Soy and Soy Milk
Lentils
Chickpeas
Most Beans
Spelt, Teff, Barley, Sorghum, Farro
Hempseed
Nuts
Green peas
Spirulina
Amaranth
Quinoa
Ezekiel Bread and other breads from "sprouted grains"
Oats and Oatmeal
Wild Rice
Chia Seeds
Nuts, Nut Butter
Broccoli, Spinach, Asparagus, Artichokes, Potatoes, Sweet Potatoes, Brussel Sprouts

PLANT BASED PROTEIN

PROTEIN PER 100G

CHICKPEAS	OATS	TOFU
7g protein	11g protein	13g protein
BROWN RICE	QUINOA	LENTILS
3g protein	4g protein	6g protein
CASHEWS	PEANUT BUTTER	ALMONDS
18g protein	28g protein	29g protein
AVOCADO	BROCCOLI	EDAMAME
2g protein	4g protein	12g protein

*Some incomplete proteins

ANIMAL BASED PROTEIN

EGGS	TURKEY MINCE	CHICKEN BREAST
14g protein	25g protein	25g protein
PRAWNS	TUNA	SALMON
18g protein	25g protein	25g protein
PORK CHOP	RIBEYE	DUCK
19g protein	19g protein	27g protein
SEMI SKIMMED MILK	GREEK YOGURT	EDAM CHEESE
4g protein	9g protein	26g protein

*All complete proteins

These vegetable sources of protein contain the most protein. The only issues may be going over on calories in order to get enough protein. Just make sure you weigh and track everything. Of course, you can always get vegetable based protein powders.

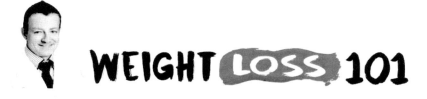

WEIGHT LOSS 101

Appendix

This section contains tons more research articles that you can read on this topic broken up into sections. I highly encourage you to read more and study more! Informed consumers are the best and most successful at health, fitness, weight loss, and life in general!

Section 1

Articles demonstrating that weight loss depends on energy balance only (calories) and that macronutrient composition does not matter at all.

Obesity Energetics: Body Weight Regulation and the Effects of Diet Composition

https://pubmed.ncbi.nlm.nih.gov/28193517/

Low Fat was actually superior to low carb. Take a look at the graph from this study.

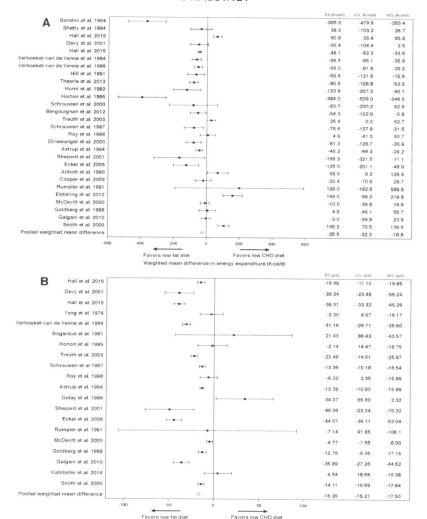

Article demonstrating that proteins and fats have a greater thermic effect of food than fat:

The Thermic Effect of Food: A Review

https://pubmed.ncbi.nlm.nih.gov/31021710/

Section 2

Articles demonstrating that while sugar intake has decreased over the years, obesity continues to rise:

Worldwide trends in dietary sugars intake

https://pubmed.ncbi.nlm.nih.gov/25623085/

Trends in dietary carbohydrate consumption from 1991 to 2008 in the Framingham Heart Study Offspring Cohort

https://pubmed.ncbi.nlm.nih.gov/24661608/

Trends in sugar-sweetened beverage consumption among youth and adults in the United States: 1999-2010

https://pubmed.ncbi.nlm.nih.gov/23676424/

Section 3

Articles demonstrating that the biggest contributor to the increase in caloric intake over the years has been fat, not sugar. Along with the graph showing the composition of diets from 1970 compared to 2010.

What's on your table? How America's diet has changed over the decades

https://www.pewresearch.org/fact-tank/2016/12/13/whats-on-your-table-how-americas-diet-has-changed-over-the-decades/

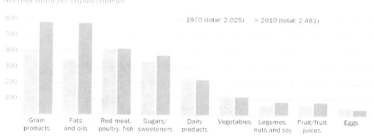

Modern American diet has gotten bigger, heavier on grains and fat

Average daily per capita calories

Section 4

Articles demonstrating that differences in glycemic load do not affect weight loss or gain when calories are equated.

Effect of Low-Fat vs Low-Carbohydrate Diet on 12-Month Weight Loss in Overweight Adults and the Association With Genotype Pattern or Insulin Secretion: The DIETFITS Randomized Clinical Trial

https://pubmed.ncbi.nlm.nih.gov/29466592/

No difference in body weight decrease between a low-glycemic-index and a high-glycemic-index diet but reduced LDL cholesterol after 10-wk ad libitum intake of the low-glycemic-index diet

https://pubmed.ncbi.nlm.nih.gov/15277154/

Metabolic and behavioral effects of a high-sucrose diet during weight loss

https://pubmed.ncbi.nlm.nih.gov/9094871/

Randomized controlled trial of changes in dietary carbohydrate/fat ratio and simple vs complex carbohydrates on body weight and blood lipids: the CARMEN study. The Carbohydrate Ratio Management in European National diets

https://pubmed.ncbi.nlm.nih.gov/11093293/

Metabolic and behavioral effects of a high-sucrose diet during weight loss

https://pubmed.ncbi.nlm.nih.gov/9094871/

The effects of four hypocaloric diets containing different levels of sucrose or high fructose corn syrup on weight loss and related parameters

https://pubmed.ncbi.nlm.nih.gov/22866961/

Section 5

Articles showing that sugar does not cause fat gain unless also accompanied by an increase in calories.

Dietary sugars and body weight: systematic review and meta-analyses of randomised controlled trials and cohort studies

Section 6

Articles demonstrating that low carb diets do not cause more weight loss than low fat/high carb diets when calories and protein are equated.

Ketogenic low-carbohydrate diets have no metabolic advantage over nonketogenic low-carbohydrate diets

https://pubmed.ncbi.nlm.nih.gov/16685046/

Energy expenditure and body composition changes after an isocaloric ketogenic diet in overweight and obese men

https://pubmed.ncbi.nlm.nih.gov/27385608/

Low carbohydrate versus isoenergetic balanced diets for reducing weight and cardiovascular risk: a systematic review and meta-analysis

https://pubmed.ncbi.nlm.nih.gov/25007189/

Section 7

Articles demonstrating that insulin levels do not predict weight gain.

The entero-insular axis and adipose tissue-related factors in the prediction of weight gain in humans

Section 8

Articles showing that overfeeding carbohydrates or fats are both equally fattening in humans.

Fat and carbohydrate overfeeding in humans: different effects on energy storage

https://pubmed.ncbi.nlm.nih.gov/7598063/

Effects of isoenergetic overfeeding of either carbohydrate or fat in young men

https://pubmed.ncbi.nlm.nih.gov/11029975/

Section 9

Article showing that NNS (non nutritive sweeteners), zero calorie sweeteners, caused more weight loss than when compared to water. Very well done study.

https://pubmed.ncbi.nlm.nih.gov/26708700/

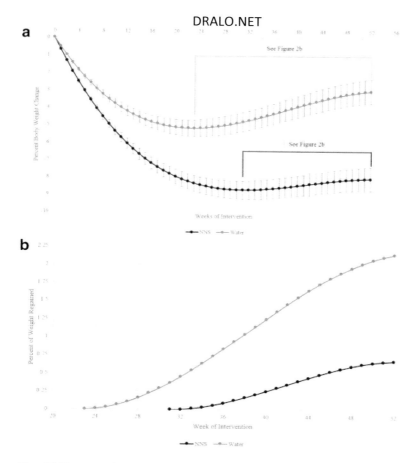

The NNS group lost more weight and kept almost all of it off.

Thank You

THE END